'For too many people, the truth about ch[...]
fying. Far from protecting them, many parents destroy their children,
emotionally, spiritually and physically. Because of the behaviour of their
'caretakers', such children grow up with violence, cruelty and the inability
to contain strong emotions structured into their psyches. Without help, these
factors can continue to wreak havoc generation after generation.

'The stories of the survivors in this book will, I hope, put the headstone
on the sort of psychiatry that explains genuine childhood experience away
as 'fantasy', dooming the person to yet another re-enactment of betrayal by
someone in authority. The violation of a child's boundaries through sexual
abuse creates immense suffering for that child, not only during the period
of abuse but later on in their life, because their spiritual, psychological and
physical boundaries lie in ruins. Such people become adults who find it
difficult to discriminate between abuse and love.

'It is essential that we tell our truth. Any book that supports this is to be
welcomed with open arms. A life lived without truth is a life devoid of
vitality—a sort of living death. Despite the enormous pain and anguish that
facing the truth fair and square causes us, it is only by doing this that we
can mourn the past and finally let it go—to embrace our lives and our
creative energies with hearts that have at last learned to love.'
Gabrielle Lord, author of *Fortress, Tooth and Claw, Jumbo, Salt, Whipping
Boy* and *Bones*

'What a joy to be included in *Breaking the Silence*. I trust it enlightens many
minds and encourages many aching hearts.'
Cathy Ann Matthews, author of *Breaking Through*

'This is the most honest book I have ever read. How well the psychological
issues are explained, without jargon. The reactions of survivors seem so
human and understandable. As a mother, I feel that all parents need this
book.'
Linda Bunch BA, MA, Reg. Psych.

'Reading *Breaking the Silence* is a totally different experience for most of us in that it recounts painful recollections of childhood. Childhood for most of us was a period of great freedom and fun, but to the people recorded in this book, childhood was a matter of anguish and inappropriate guilt.

'I believe that this book and the experiences it outlines will help a great number of people understand the difficulties and traumas with which they have grappled for much of their adult lives. It provides a way for people to see that they are not alone and through this sharing to be able to plan the future in a positive, constructive manner.

'I congratulate the editors and their authors for a very significant achievement.'

Dr John Yu, Chief Medical Officer, Westmead Children's Hospital

'Out of the darkness into the light: that's the only way to describe how I felt when I made my personal commitment to myself, to admit that I was a survivor. Admitting the truth to myself was that 'first step' that is so hard to take. Of course, once you take that first step, you realise that, like most of the 'too hard' things in life, it really isn't something we should fear as much as we do or did. Fear is the real enemy, not that first step. But, as we know, us survivors, fear is something we've been coping/living with all or most of our lives. Fear has robbed us of much of the joy that life has to offer. To fully enjoy and benefit from life we must rid ourselves of fear.

'Fear is the slavemaster, and lies are tools of repression. Fear makes a prisoner of us all. So we must find a way to free ourselves from this fear, we must seek comfort in one another's arms. For we suffered and yet we survive, so we know we are 'birds of a feather'.

'Tell the truth and you will be free. Live a lie and you are a prisoner.

'Take that first step from the world of shadows into the world of sunshine. Take that first step and set yourself free. Take that first step and walk beside me . . . I am your friend.'

Angry Anderson

Breaking the Silence

SURVIVORS OF CHILD ABUSE SPEAK OUT

EDITED BY LIZ MULLINAR & CANDIDA HUNT

Hodder & Stoughton

A Hodder & Stoughton book

First published in Australia and New Zealand in 1997 by
Hodder Headline Australia Pty Limited
(A member of the Hodder Headline Group)
10–16 South Street, Rydalmere NSW 2116

Reprinted 1997

Published in association with Belladonna Books
39 Palmer Street, Balmain NSW 2041

National Library of Australia Cataloguing-in-Publication data

Breaking the silence: survivors of child abuse speak out

ISBN 0 7336 0483 8

1. Child abuse – Case studies. 2. Adult child abuse victims – Case studies. I. Mullinar, Liz.
II. Hunt, Candida.

362.764

Cover design by Liz Seymour
Typeset by Midland Typesetters, Maryborough, Victoria
Printed in Australia by Griffin Press, Adelaide, South Australia

Contents

Acknowledgements

This book would not have been possible without the help of all ASCA members and many supporters. In particular, we would like to thank those people who volunteered to compile a chapter, which involved reading all the submitted material and putting it in some cohesive order. We acknowledge and thank: Robert Kovacs, Alison Stowes, Dr Brent Waters, Melinda Witt, Linda Honey, Rowena Robinson, Phoenix Van Dyke, Samantha Lee, Veronica Taylor, Evelyn Miers, Chris Thomson, Lisa Foster and of course ASCA's office manager, Jacqui Manning, who also managed all the coordinating. Phillipa Brennan not only compiled a chapter but also bravely did all the sorting and liaising of the material. Rod Phillips, apart from compiling a chapter, is also the chair of ASCA and Liz Mullinar's husband, so a huge extra load fell on his shoulders. Lynn Rogers from Melbourne helped compile the further reading list. Finally, a big thank you to Heather MacRae, who helped on a voluntary basis not only in the ASCA office throughout 1996 but also with the coordination work on this book.

A note about names
Most contributors to this book have used their real names. Some have used only their first names—not because they wish to be anonymous for themselves but because they are unable at this point to publicly tell of their abuse. For some, this is because the offender has acknowledged the abuse and is now trying to heal. For others, it is out of respect for the non-offending family members. For a few, it has been necessary to use a pseudonym for legal reasons. We thank all the contributors for having the bravery to speak at all.

A note about royalties
All royalties payable on sales of this book will go to Advocates for Survivors of Child Abuse, a registered charity.

Introduction

'And you will know the truth, and the truth will set you free.'
St John

There are many assumptions about child abuse prevalent today. People assume that child abuse is rare; that all child abuse is sexual; that only girls are victims; that only men are perpetrators; that ritual abuse does not exist; that what happened long ago no longer matters.

All such assumptions are false. The falsehoods have gained credence because survivors of child abuse have until now remained silent. Now, at last, members and supporters of ASCA have had the courage to break the silence. This book has been written by adult survivors of child abuse, people who have found the courage to write about their personal experience. In doing so, we hope to help other survivors find the path to healing.

All child abuse is abhorrent. As children we are dependent, inexperienced, vulnerable, trusting, sensitive. Any kind of abuse we suffer as children has a profound effect on the way we think and feel about ourselves, about other people, and about the world around us. We carry our childhood beliefs with us into adulthood; these beliefs have a huge and enduring impact on our lives.

Liz and Candida are both survivors. When Liz, in Australia, was recovering her memories and was in the depths of her pain, her sister Lucy in England mentioned Liz's plight to her friend, Candida, who had also recovered memories. Candida sat up late that night and wrote to Liz—although they had never met—to share her own experiences of a similar stage of healing.

When Liz received Candida's letter she cried for two days, because someone else understood her pain. It was the first time she discovered that she was not alone. It was so valuable for her own healing that it made her realise the unique importance of survivors to each other's healing. The discovery eventually led to the formation of ASCA and the compilation of this book. (Candida's letter to Liz is reproduced in Appendix 6, page 326.)

Liz's and Candida's childhood experiences had been very different. Liz's family life was normal, but she had two experiences of being raped, at ages 5 and 14. Both were totally forgotten, but of course they profoundly affected Liz's childhood and behaviour. Candida grew up in an emotionally dysfunctional family, was physically punished as a child, and suffered a single episode of severe sexual abuse when very young.

In other words, we have both been through the painful acknowledgement of what happened to us as children, and have experienced for ourselves the long, hard path towards healing.

A survivor of child abuse almost always grows up with a deep-felt sense of isolation. 'I can tell no one, reach out to no one, and no one can understand where I am and how I feel.' These feelings are carried through into adult life. To recognise your own feelings in the accounts of more than a hundred other survivors will, we hope, break down the wall of isolation and silence, and enable you to realise that there are others like yourself. You are not alone.

We believe that there is one essential ingredient for healing: we need to recognise and feel our pain. This means giving up denial, accepting the truth, acknowledging that we were abused as children and that it hurt, and that what was done to us was wrong and bad. The earlier you acknowledge and face the pain within you, the faster your healing will be.

It is your courage that has brought you to the stage of looking at this book. It is your courage that will allow you to begin to consider embracing the truth about your childhood. It is your courage that will enable you to move forward.

Breaking the Silence does not contain psychological theories or explanations, nor is it a self-help manual telling you what you should do, with exercises and rules for healing. We are not therapists, and don't pretend to be. We do both have a passionate belief in the human capacity for healing, and because we have travelled a similar path to yours, feel we have something to offer as companions on your healing journey. As survivors, all of us can offer each other a unique kind of validation and help.

It can be extraordinarily hard to embark on this process of acknowledging, feeling and healing. It takes such courage to rethink our past; how can we be sure it will be worth the pain? We have survived, lived, had children, managed all right, haven't we? For some the decision is easier: there is no alternative. Our lives have been so burdened with pain that we have had almost no experience of happiness, love, peace or sense of freedom, and we find it difficult even to imagine such a state of well-being. But for all people who have been abused as children, healing is possible and incredibly rewarding. With courage, patience, and loving help, no matter how bad the abuse, you can heal. It does, however, take time. If you have a bad accident or a physical illness, you accept that your body needs skilled care, that you must rest, that the healing process is at work and will take what time it needs. The same is true for minds and spirits.

We don't pretend it is easy. This is a journey full of grieving, of crying, of pain. We have to mourn everything we have lost, everything that was stolen from us, everything we never had. Many of us have spent so many years not daring to feel the way we need to feel that our pent-up emotions seem overwhelming. But the grieving period cannot be speeded up; it must be allowed to take its course. A mood at a time, a day at a time . . . and one day, you will come through.

If you're out in a boat and see a storm coming up, you have a choice. You can try to escape the storm by sailing away from it— though it will continue to pursue you—or you can turn and sail into the wind. The storm may buffet you, but if you sail through it you will eventually emerge in calm waters. As you battle with your own personal storm, we very much hope that you will be helped on your journey by reading the stories of the survivors in this book. This is a book to reach out for in the middle of the night when the pain seems unbearable and the isolation absolute.

Remember, however lonely you may feel, you are not alone. Thousands of other people all over Australia, all over the world, have felt or are feeling as you do. This is an attempt by a group of us to reach out to you, to tell you that there are companions to walk with you on your journey.

May you find healing and peace.

Liz Mullinar and Candida Hunt
1997

CHAPTER ONE

◆

Acknowledging childhood abuse

'The truth about our childhood is stored up in our body, and although we can repress it, we can never alter it. Our intellect can be deceived, our feelings manipulated, our perceptions confused, and our body tricked with medication. But someday the body will present its bill, for it is as incorruptible as a child who, still whole in spirit, will accept no compromises or excuses, and it will not stop tormenting us until we stop evading the truth.'

Alice Miller, *Thou Shalt Not Be Aware*

We hope that many of you reading this book are doing so because you already know that your childhood abuse is reflected in how you are behaving, feeling and thinking now. You might have always remembered being abused, and feel, 'If I could have one night of not remembering, one night away from the pain and the unhappiness, what a relief it would be'. Some people, however, find that well into an apparently successful adult life they begin to get an inkling that something unpleasant happened to them when they were children.

Most of us lie somewhere between these two extremes, so there is no absolutely clear distinction between the accounts in the first two sections of this chapter. Some people have always remembered everything; some recall the feelings but not the events; others the events themselves but not the feelings associated with them; others remember nothing until an event in their life triggers the memories. At any stage on the road to recovery, more memories or more details of existing memories may emerge.

Almost any abusive event in a child's life will have been accompanied by fear; most will have felt shame, bewilderment, confusion, and a host of other emotions. Some abuse—particularly some kinds of sexual abuse, which may have produced sexual arousal in the victim—may also have felt pleasurable.

When we are young, the thinking part of us is not yet very highly developed. Children feel much more immediately than adults, who tend to filter experience through thinking processes. When we begin to deal with our memories—whether this involves acknowledging what we have always known, focusing on what we have half known and tried not to think about, or exploring old events in recovered memories—sooner or later we will experience the strength and intensity of the feelings of the child we were. All feelings are valid; there is shame in none of them other than the shame imposed on us by our abusers—and that rightly belongs with the abusers, not with us.

We have included a section on the false memory myth. Advocates for Survivors of Child Abuse (ASCA) was founded as a direct result of media coverage of the false memory 'debate'. We feel as strongly as all other survivors about this issue, which can threaten our healing unless we challenge it. Those of us who have been through the extraordinary process of recovering memories, of working through the experiences they lay bare and the feelings accompanying them, know with a terrible certainty that we could not have invented them. The truth they reveal is often so horrible that at times we wish we could believe an alternative explanation—but there is none.

Those of us who have always remembered what was done to us may feel marginalised as a result of the focus on recovered memories. We too may find it hard to confront the truth: not, perhaps, wondering whether what we know happened really did take place, but doubting whether it had as great an impact as we believe. Are we just 'making a fuss', 'trying to get attention', 'inadequate and unable to cope', 'wallowing in self-pity' or 'revengeful'? There are so many labels that deny the reality of our pain. Those who have always remembered find it difficult to accept that anyone could forget a trauma which has so destroyed their life.

It was said that when the Chinese bound the feet of their girl children, the process was so painful that each pair of tiny feet was gained at the cost of 'a bucket of tears'. When, in a new era of enlightenment, these women's feet were finally released, the pain of the unbinding equalled the original pain, and the cost of freedom was again 'a bucket of tears'. We should honour the courage of all those survivors who confront the pain of unbinding their past, whether they have always remembered what happened to them or whether they are regaining their memories. It is a terrible experience, but the reward is freedom.

'I COULD NEVER FORGET'

Survivors who have always had conscious memories of abuse have no respite. We have lived in full awareness of our experiences. Because of what we were told we may believe that we deserved what happened to us, that it was our own fault. We may try to blot out the pain that haunts us, or we may feel crippled by it.

I have not forgotten anything they did to me—and often I wish I could. I want to forget the unspeakable fear, isolation and humiliation that characterised the years I lived with those known as my parents. I feel I'm starting to turn those negatives into good things—that I didn't turn out the way I am because of my parents, but in spite of them.

Jacqueline Frajer

◆

My memory of sexual abuse at the age of three has always remained clear. For some strange reason it appeared that a little boy being sexually abused by his teenage girl babysitter was nowhere near as bad as the opposite would be. I was constantly reminded of what had happened, as it became a family joke. My father (he and my mother walked in on the episode) would tell friends as I was growing up that I had had my first 'root' at three. By my late teens even I was amused ... in public. In private I didn't understand the strange and confusing feelings around this.

The big thing for me has been that until you confront the abuse it keeps affecting all areas of your life, all your relationships. I can't forget and it just won't go away.

Taylor Shane

◆

I have never had any respite from what I know. I'm not sure how young I was when it started—my first clear experiences of what happened when I was six or seven feel sickeningly familiar, so I think I must have been very young when it all began. Puberty was a nightmare for me, as I already knew things that I could not understand. As my sexuality awakened I was so horrified that whole parts of me shut down. At the age of 30 I am still struggling to regain them. My first sexual fantasies were of people in my own family; I felt so ashamed about those dreams that for a long time I wasn't able to tell anyone about them.

When I fell in love at 16 my father punished me incessantly, and some of the worst battles of my life began. As my boyfriend continued to love me—respecting my wish for an 'arm's length' relationship—my father became angry with him and started to punish him as well. Luckily, despite this I still married him. We have been together for eleven years and he still loves and respects me. What a wonderful man.

I always knew that my life was not right, but thought that people would not believe me. I tried to ask for help, but no one intervened—certainly not my school, and when I reached out for help from a counselling line the telephone counsellor on shift told me that I sounded like I came from a good home and to go home. I took my distorted beliefs about myself into adulthood. I had learnt it was not safe to be angry, so I suppressed it. When I met people who had 'recovered memories' of their traumas I was jealous. I know this sounds awful, but I thought it would be great to believe even for just a little while that these things didn't happen to me, to have even one day when I didn't wonder how I could have stopped my father, and to have some respite from what was initially guilt and is now an anger so great I wonder how it fits inside me. I have never had an identity that didn't include these experiences: there is nothing to fall back on, I don't know what it is like to feel whole. This sounds self-pitying, but I am so angry at what was taken from me again and again. I was robbed over and over.

I always felt such shame, that somehow the actions of others were a reflection of my quality as a person. The secrets and the hiding became a part of my life, so that even now when I am afraid I automatically assume I will get into trouble, and try to make up a story to protect myself. Usually I don't give in to this any more, but the thoughts and the fear are still there.

Wendy Stamp

◆

I have always known about the abuse inflicted on me by my cousin, but apart from having a deep sense of shame and guilt about it, I believed for a long time that it didn't affect my life in the present—and more than that, that I was responsible for it because I was ten years old when it started and I 'should' have been able to say 'no', run away, or tell someone.

I started therapy for issues of depression, and spent the first year with my therapist dealing with the pain I felt about my parents' lack of love and care of me. At the beginning of my second year of counselling, the sexual abuse issue came up, and I promptly told my counsellor, 'My sexual relationship with my husband is fine. The abuse from my cousin hasn't affected me.' (I didn't want to look at it because the shame was so overwhelming, and I felt too scared to admit some of the feelings I had in case he thought I was crazy.) He suggested I should join a group for survivors of childhood sexual abuse run by one of his colleagues. I went along more because I trusted his judgement than because I thought I needed to.

At the beginning of the first eight-week term I was terrified, but by the end of it I felt safe and accepted, and I realised they weren't going to pressure me to say or do anything I wasn't ready for. I went back for another three terms. The group helped me normalise my feelings and the denial about the abuse. I stopped believing I was crazy and was finally able to start looking at the issues with my therapist.

The next four months were overwhelming and fearful as I 'went back' emotionally to the place of abuse and acknowledged the pain of that little girl who was terrified and alone and unable to stand up for herself . . . and I began the process of learning to love her again.

I went and spent some time in a Sunday school class full of ten-year-old girls at a friend's church. They were so young and innocent. It was important for me to realise that I really was still such a baby at the age of ten.

Stephanie Mitchell

◆

Because I can clearly recall everything that happened to me, I tend to project my horrific memories onto everything I do. In my isolation, loneliness, fear and anger I felt like some kind of freak—as far as I could see, other kids didn't have the same violence in their homes that I had to put up with. When I was about ten I went to a friend's house and felt the difference in the atmosphere as soon as I walked in: it was full of warmth and love.

The crunch came when my friend's father came home. All the kids were delighted to see him, and he was just as glad to see them. He was interested in their lives and openly affectionate to them and to his wife. I was aghast. I thought it was normal to be afraid of your father, and to hate him. That visit confirmed for me that something was very wrong in my little world. I didn't feel there was anyone I could talk to about living with a violent father and a mother who stood by watching it all happen and doing nothing.

I feel angry that the events of my childhood still influence me so much. They don't run my life as much as they used to, but I often still do something because I know my parents wouldn't approve, and that's not a good reason. I would really like to do just one thing without wondering what their reaction would be.

Jacqueline Frajer

✦

I am a young man of 31, married with two children. That sounds normal enough, but I don't consider myself normal. I have always struggled with life and living . . .

I don't know how many times I was raped, and to be honest I don't really want to know. My memories go as far back as I can remember, and involve both my mother and my father. As a child I suffered in isolation, and now I continue to suffer isolation. Only I can know the deprivation and utter filth I experienced at the hands of my own parents. I never really forgot or repressed what happened to me, but I did sit on the big picture for a long time. It wasn't until I began to disclose that the details started flowing and filling in the jigsaw of my life. There isn't a part of my life that hasn't been touched by what they did to me.

David Patterson

✦

My father was a charismatic figure in his sphere of influence, everybody's friend, a solid citizen given to helping those less fortunate than himself, and no doubt seen as a 'good father, a good provider' for his family of four girls. Growing up it seemed to us that our parents were rather punitive, restrictive and apparently uncaring. The rod was certainly not spared. Children were to be seen and not heard, and if present at all we were not to speak unless spoken to. When it was necessary to be seen it was preferable to be smiling and wearing a pretty dress.

My overwhelming memory of childhood is of being unhappy, seeming to live life at a tangent from the rest of the family, desperate to conform to the family 'norms' but never quite measuring up, however hard I tried. I felt unwanted and unloved. I was convinced I was a bad, stupid and ugly child, and it seemed obvious to me that I was the one with the problem. These messages were constantly reinforced in my hearing. It was not until I left home at 20 I began to realise I was an intelligent, creative and gifted young woman. This knowledge is difficult to hang onto, and yet it continues to challenge the well-scripted messages I believed for so many years.

Barb Storey

◆

My childhood family always lived geographically and socially isolated. My mother would go off to work, and my unemployed father would keep me home on the pretence of having to work on the farm. He was a violent man with a lightning-trigger temper; I cannot remember a time when I wasn't afraid of him.

I don't remember him threatening me if I told anyone of his sexual abuse of me, but I knew what he was capable of—attacking me with whips, firing bullets at me, throwing knives at me, depriving me of food: he used all these tactics, and more. I remember him taking me, naked, into his bed and the smell and texture of the bedclothes. Later I remember him watching me as I crouched over an enamel bowl washing my private parts. But I don't remember what happened between the bed and the bowl.

During therapy I've discovered that I had learned to 'blank out' when events or emotions become too uncomfortable to deal with. For years I thought it was daydreaming or that I was getting early onset Alzheimer's. People have often accused me of not listening, and at times I have found myself in strange places, unable to recall how I got there. (Recently I've observed that my dissociative periods are lessening in frequency and length.)

I often experience 'body pain', such as severe anal and lower abdominal pain, when I talk of the abuse. Loss of libido and body pain after sex with my long-term, very loving and caring husband, are still problems for me, and I still have frequent nightmares.

Grace Power

◆

Having experienced memories of abuse from both sides—some that I always remembered and others that I have recovered—it has been my experience that even when a memory is not repressed it is nevertheless suppressed, pushed to a place where it is at least not thought about. Another thing I found is that where the pictorial memory is not forgotten, the feelings often are.

I clearly remember being subjected to daily oral rape by a baby-sitter's adult son for a time when I was only four. There were other, later, assaults, and extensive physical abuse by my parents. I remembered these events, but I forgot completely how it felt, maintaining until I was in my early twenties that it 'hadn't affected me' even though I was suicidally depressed (anger turning inwards) and had been in abusive relationships (expecting no better).

I was taken completely by surprise at the extent of the fear, anger and pain I found as I rescued my inner children from these terrible places. I truly think that at the time I had no other option. I did try to tell my mother when I was four what was being done to me. She was angry with me, so I learnt that it was better to keep such things to myself. I was never able to eat an ice cream when I was young without pangs of sickness, because the abuser would liken the oral rape to eating them. As for the physical abuse, this was accepted by me as part of life.

Working with the abuse I've always remembered is probably easier than trying to reclaim lost memories. I've found that it is also possible to forget part of an experience. For example, I remember (and always have) being assaulted when I was 11 by a man who then assaulted a friend of mine in my presence. I know, intellectually, that he abused her after me, but I cannot remember exactly what took place—and I think that's the nature of shock.

As I've said, I can remember what happened to me when I was four, but I did not remember until quite recently that this man also attempted on one occasion to penetrate me, desisting only when the pain made me scream.

I find I still become angry when I think about the fact that one of my earliest memories is of having a penis in my mouth. I'm entitled to that sense of outrage; I value that dear little girl.

Louise Plummer

✦

I have always known, always remembered, but I never told anyone. I never thought of it as a secret, but I knew that to tell anyone would mean certain death for me or—worse—the disbanding of my entire family. What a huge responsibility for a little girl.

Sexual abuse—the words really don't sound that bad. Sex is a normal part of everyday life and often a very enjoyable part, but when an adult forces his sexual depravity on a child of four then the crime is the most disgusting, degrading and dehumanising breach of trust.

The pain, hurt, anguish and shame go all the way through to the four-year-old's soul. I was 'intensively' injured but couldn't or wouldn't feel the emotions. I was 20 before I had the courage to stop the abuse.

Sixteen years of pain, fear, mistaken love, self-loathing and self-hate have all permeated my soul. This is where the emotions sat for another 22 years, until at the age of 42 I finally found the voice to tell the world of the pain and terror I experienced for all those years.

Carmol Morley

✦

I always knew I had been emotionally abused as a child. What I did not know until recently, at the age of 50, was that the way my mother treated me—physically and emotionally—came under the heading of child sexual abuse. Over the years I had tried to describe what had been done to me to several psychiatrists, but until now no one had the courage to 'speak the unspeakable' and tell me the truth. Once my truth had been recognised, I was able to confirm it, first in a book by Joel Covitz called *Emotional Child Abuse: The Family Curse* and later in other writings.

I was stunned by the knowledge that I had minimised, with the help of my previous therapists, such damaging and destructive behaviour that I had later almost killed myself. Much worse was my own shame in not recognising the full extent of other children's abuse while working with abused children as a doctor for a few years. My excuse is that this was 12 to 15 years ago! So much more is known now; then I had no one who could truly help me to accept my own situation.

As I write this I am only three months into my therapy with my 'enlightened witness', as Alice Miller would say, so I am unable to tell you that I always knew everything. On the contrary, I am convinced that there are other memories I have forgotten, which I may or may not recover. Time will tell.

Sarah McGregor

◆

RECOVERING MEMORIES

The debate surrounding recovered memories is a tortured one. The idea that such an immense experience could ever be lost to consciousness can be hard to believe. However, it is absurd to suggest that there are hundreds of therapists deliberately attempting to implant memories in the minds of their clients. The proof of the truth in the process of recovering memories lies in the fact that it leads to our healing. Our minds may be capable of confusion, lies and fantasies, but bodies cannot lie.

Almost all of us who have suffered serious abuse have felt 'body memories' in which recurring pain or sensations insist on reminding us of early abuse. This pain miraculously disappears once we have remembered the abuse, as does our emotional pain such as sleeplessness and depression. A false memory would not lead to such healing. Our own bodies remind us that what we remember is the truth. The most injurious effect on our healing is an accusation that the hell we are going through is false or imagined. We know what we know—and no one should take that away from us.

It is widely believed that the recovery of memories is a phenomenon that takes place almost exclusively in therapy, and only in relation to claims of sexual abuse. Some say that there is no real evidence for the truth of these memories and no psychological mechanisms to account for them. It is also claimed that it would be impossible to forget such trauma.

Recent research disputes all these premises. Therapy is the least commonly reported cue for the return of traumatic memories, and the experience of delayed memory is not restricted to survivors of sexual abuse. With delayed memories of abuse it is just as possible to find corroborative evidence as it is with remembered abuse. And studies worldwide have come up with remarkably consistent figures on the prevalence of disrupted memories for abuse: in a Canadian study 61% of people surveyed did not always remember their abuse, in a Dutch study 57% and in a US study 64%. In another US study, interviews with a hundred women whose sexual abuse had resulted in hospital treatment when they were children found that as adults 17 years later 38% of them claimed never to have been sexually abused. Australian statistics tell a similar story. In ASCA's July 1996 survey of survivors, 55% did not always remember their abuse. Of these, more than half recovered memories before receiving any professional help.

While the professionals debate repression, suppression and dissociative conditions, and the media report only what they choose, as survivors we know that the process called 'forgetting' takes place to protect our vulnerable and overwhelmed child from the full horror of an agonising experience.

So how do repressed memories return to our consciousness? They come as experiences detached from meaning, flashes of image without cause, nightmares without apparent foundation, tastes, sounds and bodily sensations without stimulus, fears and uncontrollable feelings. And all the old demons of our childhood return: self-hatred, despair, self-accusation. No accuser could equal the ferocity with which most survivors at first reject their own memories.

When we begin to recover memories many of us think we must be going crazy. How could these strange—often terrifying or obscene—scenes in our heads be real if we did not remember them? The way memory works is still not fully understood, but as survivors we understand enough to know that we would not wish on an enemy, let alone on ourselves (however bad we fear we may be) the difficulties we experience as the memories surface.

Recovering memories is hell. It would have to be the most desolate experience of a lifetime. He is dead, and I feel as if I have the life sentence.

Eloise Kaitlin

◆

Two and a half years ago now my life really started to change. Suddenly everything I knew about myself, my parents, my family and my place in the world was very murky. The grip and control I had on my life started to slip. Looking back, I now know that the defences and controls I had put in place as a child were starting to wear thin. I could move no further behind that protective barrier, for large holes had begun to expose me, leaving me vulnerable.

Until I started therapy two years ago I had kept up such a brave face. I had been such a good child, student and worker. I thought I had made it; I had always thought, 'Just get to be an adult and it will be okay'. I thought I was going to be able to make it and leave my wretched life behind me.

I finished my Masters course and began my professional working life as a psychologist. I met and married a wonderful person. I felt I had my morals and political perspectives worked out; I knew right from wrong; I was dependable; I had a number of friendships.

But a chain of events in my working life and personal life, including my marriage and the death of my mother's mother, with whom I had always been close, triggered an incredible dis-ease and rockiness within me. I tried to soldier on, but was unable to with-stand the 'falling apart' feeling. I was no longer in control. At times I was paranoid. I was tired, became sick easily, and had chronic infections. That was the start of piecing together and consciously realising that I had been sexually abused by my father, who had had sole custody of me since I was 18 months old. It was also the start of grieving for my mother, from whom I had been separated all my life. At times she lived in mental institutions, until she suicided when I was 12.

I guess that was when I started to 'recover memories'. At the time I thought I was just crazy, with a sick imagination. At first it was just uncomfortable feelings and thoughts about my father. The sexual nature of these scared me. I thought I had some sick sexual fantasy or attachment. I dreamed of accusing him and telling my family that I had been sexually abused. I always discounted or minimised these messages, refusing to recognise that they had any significance. But they persisted, until I finally asked myself, 'Is it possible that this really did happen?'

I was to move back and forth many times before I actually started to piece together the signs. Even today I'm an expert at doubting my reality, and go through periods of discounting these signs.

It is still so very hard for me to fully understand the process that I have been through over the last two years. I think that recalling, thinking about, talking about traumatic events in our lives will always in itself be traumatic to some extent, especially in the initial stages. To me the healing, the therapeutic value, depends on how we ourselves and others react to this process. When it is handled sensitively and appropriately the trauma passes, just as it does in the grieving process.

Eva Gordon

◆

At the age of five I was lured away from a park, where I was playing with my brothers, by a man I didn't know. He made friends with me and then tied me up, threatened me violently and sexually assaulted me. At the time it was thought best never to mention the assault to me again, and let me just forget about it. My mother was advised not to lay any charges, and none ever were laid, even though the police had identified the man. My mother never spoke of it again, even though I asked her about it when I was 13 and memories of the event began to resurface. I thought it was a dream that I was having over and over again. I wondered why a dream could be so complete in every detail. For a long time, I thought that I might be crazy because the dream and the nightmares were so consistent. At that time I also began to wet the bed and suffer other illnesses. Still my family never spoke of the assault.

During my teenage years my self-esteem suffered dreadfully. I became sexually inappropriate: I was extremely promiscuous in an effort to please everyone and be liked. I began to drink alcohol at that time and had sex with everybody. My body became much larger for no reason—I don't remember eating more. I had been very bright and achieved many good things in my very early years, but by the time I entered high school I was uninterested in school and made little effort to achieve academically.

Elizabeth Quinn

◆

The dictionary definition of repressed memory goes like this: repress—force a painful or undesirable memory from the conscious mind into the unconscious mind; memory—the ability to remember, retain or recall what is learned or experienced. If you ask survivors to give our own definition of repressed memory, you will probably hear words like horror, nightmare, craziness, unbelievable, traumatic, painful, evil, mistake and many more.

I have spent 11 years reliving my childhood abuse, and I have used all these words many times with many different feelings. Unfortunately there is no way you can be prepared for the emotions and the confusion you will experience with memory recall. There is no way of knowing the questions you will ask yourself over and over again, the numerous times you will argue with yourself and accuse yourself of creating the things you are remembering. There is no way of knowing how you are going to cope with the denial from yourself and other people, the feelings of being alone, of having no one to turn to.

Haven't we travelled this road before? Didn't we experience all these feelings and fears many years ago? Yes, we certainly did; the feelings are familiar. (There is a difference, though: now we are not alone. There are many people who want to help us have a voice and an identity. We have turned the corner, and we are no longer 'victims'—we are 'survivors'.)

Reliving my childhood abuse was not easy, and most of the time I truly thought I was crazy. I thought I was possessed by some evil spirit, or maybe I was evil myself. I must have been evil because of what my family did to me—it never occurred to me that maybe they were the evil ones. I have experienced the self-destructive measures we take when the pain becomes too much to bear. I have kept myself in denial because it was too hard to accept that my family could violate me the way they did.

When my solicitor handed me court records that substantiated my recall, several days passed before I could look at them because I did not want to believe and face the horrible truth. I have now accepted and confronted the facts and have given myself permission to grieve. Yes, I have finally grieved for the innocent childhood I will never know. At times the anger returns, but I now have the freedom to get to know myself and to give some love and understanding to that little girl who still lives deep inside me.

Joan Edgar

◆

I had absolutely no idea that my past held a ghastly secret until my memories began to make their way into my conscious mind. The way I led my life had given me no clues about the fact that for 20 years I had suppressed the knowledge of several years of father-daughter rape. I had studied to tertiary level, travelled, married and had a child I loved dearly. It was his birth and, some months later, the death of my father that seemed to set off my subconscious time bomb.

The first sign of something strange was the way my anxiety level and inner tension suddenly increased for no obvious reason. Then one day during a visualisation exercise led by a psychic healer I discovered a picture of myself as a child, and immediately I knew. It was as though a door had opened and I could see all the way back. My body felt ten tonnes lighter. I soon began to change as I confronted a range of memories. The fact that I had concealed my past from myself so successfully, and my lack of emotional symptoms or unexplained illness, caused me to question not only my recovered memories but also myself as a person. I struggled for a long time with the idea that I might have been making them all up, despite the recurring theme of abuse in the memories that surfaced, and the obvious improvement in my physical state and my outlook on life as I dealt with them. It was to be some years before I found the right kind of people to help me confront the visions and emotions from my past and free myself from it.

Angela R.

◆

Most of my recovered memories are of feelings. I had so many memory 'photographs', but they were merely images. They were clear and precise, and always with me. Other images would flash in and out of the 'movie theatre' of my mind, yet seldom stay long enough to be identified. These were hard to handle. They haunted me because I couldn't hold them. To recover the memories I had to identify the feelings, which had no pictures, and these feelings were mortally dangerous to me.

The feelings came back when I recovered further memories, the ones I had squashed out of my mind altogether. Now I have feelings, pictures and combinations of the two. I believe that the pain in my body (chronic fatigue syndrome) is the physical manifestation of the emotional pain I was never allowed to feel as a child.

Linley Valente

◆

I have always known that I was abused, but there were some things I did not remember at all until I recovered the memories. Every time this happened it was sudden, unexpected and came out of the blue. In some ways these new memories have been harder to cope with than what I'd always remembered, I think because the feelings are so intense when the memory comes back. One of the worst memories returned when my daughter was 18 months old; it was of abuse I had suffered when I was the same age. The intensity of the feelings was so powerful that at the time I didn't think I would ever recover.

Juley Taben

◆

There are certain classic ways in which memories of abuse can surface. I found the pressure in my life weakening my ability to repress the past. Even an examination by a doctor or dentist could trigger a frightening onslaught of memories, of feelings. Some other memories began to emerge in the form of psychosomatic pains.

Margaret Wood

◆

I am the only daughter of a middle-class family. This would guarantee me a life of opportunities, or so I was led to believe. Unfortunately, I was also the daughter of a chronic alcoholic, drug abuser and food abuser, with manic depression. All of which—in my experience—goes hand in hand with child abuse.

At the age of 21, I entered my recovery—the recovery of myself and my childhood, though I didn't know it at the time. I entered a 12-step programme called Overeaters Anonymous. What does this have to do with recovered memories? Everything, because I discovered that food wasn't my problem, it was my friend. During my childhood food had kept me alive to allow me to get to this point in my life, where I can share my experiences, my strength and my hope in healing.

I entered my recovery with virtually no childhood memories, good or bad. I had completely blocked most of my childhood through the use of food and other coping mechanisms. I thought this was normal, but as I put food aside and started to write, many memories came back. At first most were fairly safe memories, ones with only slight discomfort, I believe, because that is all I could cope with. This was an exciting process for me because I could feel parts of me fitting into place like a jigsaw puzzle. However, over time my memories became more and more clear and more and more painful. Thank God I had developed a supportive network of other people who were also in their own healing.

What came out of later stages in my healing was such a shock to me. I had had no idea of my true history. I cannot deny any of what came up for me because of the intensity and the pain. The floodgates were finally opened. My body had stored the energy of the abuse, and with the commitment I had made my mind and body started releasing the memories. At times I would lie in a foetal position and couldn't move. At times I couldn't breathe, and I became completely immobilised. At other times I would just start screaming and felt as though I couldn't stop. At the end of each healing session I felt totally drained and so vulnerable. It was like being stripped of armours that I had held dear to me for so long. But with each healing I could feel myself become stronger and more empowered.

Unfortunately, at the time there were a lot of accusations of false memories being bandied around the media, and members of my own family also made me feel as though I had false memories. Thank God I was sure that no one could make up the kind of pain that was coming out of my body, mind and soul. Although I became extremely sensitive and vulnerable, and needed to protect myself, I knew that it was true.

Deane Griffin

◆

When the horror surfaced I had an immense feeling of relief. Why? Because for the first time my life started to make sense. Everything that had puzzled me fell into place with startling clarity. We have to endure our trauma twice: once at the time, and again during the reliving of those experiences. Both are of equal intensity, and need incredible fortitude to survive.

Margaret Wood

◆

Initially I entered therapy to work on abuse of which I had always been aware. One afternoon, about a year into therapy, I was sitting evaluating my healing so far. I was feeling a bit odd, when suddenly I felt a tremendous cold, and a slimy feeling like someone licking my body. I could smell gas and see blue walls. I began to scream, with part of my mind trying to regain control.

I had a horrible anxiety attack that lasted three days. I didn't know there was a name for what I was experiencing, so I assumed I'd gone mad.

This process was quite spontaneous. I knew nothing about repressed memories, and I thought I had always remembered my abuse. I can categorically state that there was never anything 'suggested' or 'implanted'.

I struggled with these darkening memories for six months, and finally told my therapist, convinced that she too would think I was mad and would not want to help me any more. But she didn't think I was mad, she encouraged me to go with what was happening. In the end I had no choice, as the more I fought it the more distressing it became.

I had horrible nightmares, always feeling that there was someone standing next to my bed. I felt very out of control, and it was extremely hard to talk to anyone about the substance of these 'pictures' in my head as I felt the worst shame.

Now, seven years later, I have come to terms with the fact— yes, fact—that a close family friend raped me very brutally when I was between the ages of eight and ten. I think that working with the things I already knew in effect 'woke up' the forgotten things. Why was I able to remember some things but not others? I believe this is because the forgotten abuser was more harmful to me than the remembered abuse: each time I was raped I thought I was going to die; and I remembered these experiences in much the same way as I had originally experienced them.

Also, I loved the abuser very much, and just could not meld the 'uncle' who did these things to me with the one who sat and drank beer with Dad. Many other men abused me in later years, but I did not share the same relationship with them as I had with this one. For a while it felt as though the memories and the pain would never end, but I would like to assure everyone who is experiencing this feeling, that eventually it does end. There will come a time when you feel strong and valid, knowing the truth and no longer fearing its implications.

Louise Plummer

◆

To admit to being a survivor of incest is a tremendous step, but it is only one of many. There are so many years of painful memories to climb over that I feel if I am forever climbing mountains.

I could not remember any of this until I was very happy and content and staying with my boyfriend. Snippets of memory came back in the form of nightmares, usually in the cold dark depths of the night. I still do not know how often incidents of abuse occurred, as I have memory blanks and I am still journeying through my flashbacks, fitting them in where they belong. However, I do know that it began when I was at least three and continued until I was 17 and left home. Sometimes I think abuse is too soft a word: torture seems more appropriate.

To any other survivors, I'd say: do not fear the memories, as they cannot hurt you; and do not bury them, as they can control your life. Deal with it, as it will keep coming back until you do. Despite all the pain and sadness, anger and bitterness, humiliation, shame and despair, there is one thing greater than all of these: HOPE. Cling to it every day. If you survived the torment, you are strong and resilient enough to survive the healing. It may be a long road to travel, but it is worth it to make it into the sunshine and never have to go back into the shadows of your past.

Penny Stevens

◆

At the age of 30 I had memories of my boyhood that were mostly happy. I had vague recollections of physical abuse, but made the conscious decision to let sleeping dogs lie. I was a good corporate man who constantly preached positive thinking and to control negative emotions. (I am sure many of us males believe at some stage that most emotions are the domain of the irrational.) However, the death of my mother sent me reeling.

I tried psychoanalysis but did not get very far, so on the advice of a trusted friend I tried Gestalt therapy. Within a few weeks I was recalling specific instances of physical abuse and the pain and grief associated with this. From the age of 11 I'd been forbidden to cry—being threatened with another belting if I did. Men don't cry. In this Gestalt group my composure and intellect were moved aside to expose emotional agony and clear images of violent beatings.

I found it difficult to believe these memories were true, and tried putting them down to my imagination. When my sister verified the experiences and expressed surprise at my not remembering as clearly as she did, we discovered a fascinating phenomenon. I recalled with great clarity her beatings, and how powerless I had felt at not being able to help her, yet I forgot my own. She remembered all of my abuse and felt desperately sorry for me, but likewise had forgotten most of her own.

If you're afraid of recovered memories, please don't be. Yes, the initial confrontation is painful (and so is the process of healing), but the results are profound freedom.

Taylor Shane

◆

When I first went to see a therapist, for help with the dreadful dreams I was having, he asked me about my family history and background, and I recounted that I had had a happy, normal childhood, with caring parents. He accepted this without question, and at no time suggested that any form of abuse or childhood trauma existed in my life. His whole strategy for my therapy was to deal with what was bothering me, and to have me feeling well and happy with myself in the shortest possible time.

My life with my parents, brothers and sisters was happy, even though I 'knew' there was something wrong with me. I was different from the other kids. I never talked about these feelings because it seemed so crazy. At 19 I married my boyfriend of three years, and within three months found that I was married to a violent alcoholic. Two children and almost four years later I left him, and continually questioned myself about why I had married him in the first place. I did not fit the psychological pattern of abuse following abuse: my parents were not violent, did not drink too much and did not abuse us.

But families consist of more than one generation. I guess that my questioning, coupled with the nightmares and many little triggers, led to the return of my memories. Eventually I remembered that at the age of three I had been raped by my grandfather, who was an alcoholic and at times violent. He continued to abuse me until his death when I was eight.

On one occasion my grandmother found me semi-conscious in a pool of blood and a doctor was called. I was taken to his surgery through the back entrance so that no one would see me. I remember the doctor's face, some of the conversation, and a feeling that the doctor was angry with my grandfather, even though he assured my grandparents that I would forget it once my body had healed. I was told I must not tell anyone or 'Poppy' would go to jail. I believe my aunt nursed me and kept me with her for eight weeks. My parents were never told what had happened to me.

Elizabeth McMinn

◆

For the first 13 years of my life I was severely and sadistically abused sexually, physically and emotionally by both my mother and my father.

For another 32 years I had absolutely no memories of the abuse. I considered that I had had a normal childhood with parents who loved me and cared about my well-being. Unlike others who have repressed similar occurrences in their past, I had no years of unexplained physical or psychological illnesses. I married, had three children, worked intermittently, swam daily and competitively with AUSSI Masters, in a full and actively satisfying life. Or so I thought.

It started with a hysterectomy. I had been troubled for years with very painful periods and eventually, at the age of 45, saw a gynaecologist who diagnosed endometriosis. An abdominal growth was also found, which required the removal of my womb and one ovary. After the operation I just didn't want to come home! I didn't know why—it was just that the thought of going home made me frightened, and led to depression and bouts of tears. Everyone said, 'It's quite normal to be depressed after a hysterectomy', but that didn't account for my absolute fear of returning to my old routine. After six months of continuous abdominal pain and tests to rule out further intervention, my GP suggested hypnosis as a way of relaxing. The hypnotherapist tried his best, but something inside me fought against it—rejecting the opportunity to let my subconscious take over—and I was left in even more fear than before. He suggested that I see a psychiatrist.

That was seven years ago, and I have been uncovering my awful past bit by painful bit with the help of my therapist ever since.

The abuse was horrific. It's most likely that my mother suffered from a post-partum psychosis after my birth, and when my father started having an affair with another woman my mother blamed me. ('If I hadn't been pregnant with you he would never have done it.') At the age of three my father began sexually abusing me, using the old threat of 'If you don't let me, I'll go away and not love you'. My mother found out about this, and from that point on regarded me as 'the other woman' and treated me accordingly. My father continued his sexual activities with me until I was 13, usually with my consent and sometimes at my instigation—something I have great difficulty accepting! Did I have a choice? My intellect tells me, 'No', but I feel constant shame deep inside me about this.

I see my therapist twice a week; the sessions are painful and exhausting. I am just starting to put feelings to the memories, and am coping with such incredible terror each time. Anger is there sometimes, but it's still too threatening to be angry with anyone other than my therapist. I'm also terrified of getting better: I'll have to give her up! However, I continue to go, so something inside me must want to get through this. I'm 52 now, and at times it feels as though there's not much time left for me to 'have a life'. I guess I'll fight on, and one day it might start to hurt a little less and I'll start to live a little more. I hope so.

Jan Watson

◆

'What is frightening to me is the level of suppressed abuse and the number of people who have lived with soul-destroying memories for so long.' *Chief Inspector Fraser after Operation Paradox, Victoria, 1995.* Operation Paradox is a phone-in conducted by the police for people to give confidential information about sexual assault. It is run annually during Child Protection week.

◆

I went into therapy after months of believing I was losing my mind. I was in a mentally abusive relationship, and his threats were similiar to those of the man who abused me. I had been sexually abused three or four times a week at school by a teacher. My partner used threats to manipulate me, just as my teacher had used threats to manipulate me to do his bidding. These new threats brought old memories flooding back. For a long time I did not know if they were real—all I felt was shame that I had allowed the teacher to have his way with me. I took the blame upon myself.

Kym Dunbar

◆

I am a 28-year-old psychiatric social worker with two children. Recently my husband left me; several months before he went, I started recalling terrifying and disturbing memories from my child-hood. They involved my estranged father—and even though my mother, grandmother and my (ex) husband did not believe me, I knew without a doubt they were true. I knew that he had molested me because:

a) he had tried to do it to my two sisters;

b) he had also tried to do it again when I was 20, which I had never forgotten;

c) the feelings associated with the memories were incredibly vivid, and since then my life has fallen into place. It's as if the missing piece of the jigsaw has been found. Because of my recovered memories I lost many things: my husband, my mother, credibility in my family, trust in men ... However, the gains more than make up for this: freedom, a sense of peace, a new beginning, understanding. I no longer suffer from insomnia, depression, overeating or constant anxiety.

Jane Lewis

✦

Somewhere from deep within
a faint cry reaches out,
tentative, seeking, hurting.

Somewhere way out there
a strong wall stands,
cold, hard, rejecting.

Somewhere way out there
another stands,
loving, caring, waiting,
as though beyond the wall.

I long to listen
and to heed his call.

Yet what dark unknown pathway lies in between?
What danger lurks in hidden corners?

What gruesome thought lies waiting to devour?
Dare I face the conflict and the pain?

Written six days before Julie Waddy recovered her first memories.

◆

At about 3.30 in the morning, as I couldn't sleep, I was watching TV. A commercial came on—a little girl was yelling at this doll. She was yelling abuse at it, and as I watched the memories of my own unremembered abuse came flooding back. It was so over-whelming I felt sick, and I started crying.

Kerrie Ann Hawkins

◆

I still have difficulty coming to terms with the facts of what really happened, and to realise that I was abused as a child. I went through all the horrors of body memories, nightmares, flash-backs and fear tremors, headaches, biliousness and excruciating pain throughout my body. The sad thing is, at the time I did not understand that this was normal and thought that I was going crazy. I tried to suppress it all again because of my fear of what was going to come up next. I have always had an incredible rage inside me, and now I understand where it was all coming from.

Linda Honey

◆

At first it's only an inkling.
Flash of lights on an opaque screen.
Yet somehow . . . I know.

I disbelieve, but I know.

I get the courage. I go further.

See pictures, snapshots of pain hidden in the
    protected corners of my mind.
Tentatively working their way out.

Not to hurt me, but to heal me.

It happens again, 21 years later, though he is not there.
A body memory?
A body memory.
Now I know it's real.

Now the healing can begin.
I fight back. Kick and scream and yell, 'No!'
I am powerful.

I face him for real. Look him in the eye and
    say, 'I remember'.
His denial is like a feather in the breeze.
I toss it aside lightly—it is meaningless.
I am powerful. I am strong. I have survived.

Now I can live.

Karen I. Shanbrom

◆

Until recently the only memory of abuse I had was of when I was
11 years old and Dad got me to sit on his lap. Soon his hands
were going up and down. I felt confused and said I needed to go
to the toilet, where I stayed with the door locked for about half
an hour. When I came out I sat as far away from him as possible,
not knowing if I would be told off or reproached.

It was a small incident, but one that left me unable to have first a boyfriend, then my husband, touch me without feeling like shrivelling up inside. I am getting over it but without the patience of my husband I wouldn't have coped. At the back of my mind I knew I had been dealt with wrongly when I was much younger, so I meditated and said, 'I need to feel free'. I knew I couldn't find freedom without getting out whatever memories I had stored away. I started doing self-regression work on myself, and although I couldn't get much out I think I brought it to the surface. A few days later I was talking to someone when a drunk man came up and started asking why I wasn't talking to him, what was wrong. I felt myself shrinking inside and I had to leave.

Memories started to come flooding in from the back of my mind. I rang a friend and asked what I should do. I was advised to sit quietly under a tree until my husband got home. I did that, continually forcing back the memories. When the van pulled up and my husband got out I couldn't hold it any longer, and I cried and cried. He thought at first that I had smashed the car. I explained through my tears that I had to tell him everything that had come through.

My memories went back to when I was only a few months old, with Dad undoing my nappies. When I described the memories of what was being done to me by the time I was two years old, I was hitting my husband and screaming, 'Why did he do this to me, why?'

Regaining the memories left me feeling tired, angry and confused, and it took me weeks to feel okay and as though I could cope again. I still have trouble sitting in a bath, as the memories still come back of what happened to me between the ages of five and seven, when my father—who said he was just washing us—always sat in the bath with us.

Andrea Willis

◆

Although I was aware that my family life had not been stable or particularly happy, as a young adult I did not identify myself as a person who had been abused. My story of gradual recognition that my personal history contained abuse, and my healing, started in 1993.

I was a quiet child and teenager, studious, rather a loner. I grew up in rural NSW. After my HSC I moved away from home to study at university. When I married in 1992 we established our home in the city where I had gained my degree. Work and activities with our church friends were pretty much our life.

I was part of the group who sang at evening services at our church. At a service one day I suddenly felt upset and was aware of an almost physical cracking inside me. Tears started to well up; I hoped nobody in the congregation could sense my distress, and wasn't sure I would be able to sing the rest of the song bracket. During the next hymn I was overwhelmed, and left the church sobbing. People came outside to comfort me and to ask what was wrong. I couldn't tell them, because I didn't know myself.

The next six months were particularly difficult. I had been depressed for a few weeks before breaking apart at church, but had assumed it was just because of stress at work. Now the depression worsened, and I withdrew from everyone and stopped attending church. Concentrating at work was very hard. People knew I was in trouble, but I put off anyone who attempted to talk to my husband and me and they left us alone. One night my husband and I talked about sexual abuse, and I told him I had been abused—which was news to me too, for I had no specific memories, and I didn't really believe it, even after telling him. Some time later we attended a community information session on sexual abuse run by a Christian-based counselling organisation. As the effects on adults of childhood abuse were being described I thought, 'Yes, that's what it is like. Maybe I really have been abused.' I cried and left the room. Each time I returned to hear some more, the tears welled up and I had to leave again. We went home early. My husband, exasperated at my emotional behaviour, wouldn't talk to me. I felt confused and isolated. At that time I still had no clear idea of anything in my past that I could call abuse and so didn't seek help—I just wouldn't have known what to say.

A month later, wanting to reach out, I went to see a woman from another church who had experience in counselling people who had been sexually abused. I didn't have any memories to talk about. She talked to me about sexual abuse and the effects it has on children and on adults. When she asked me about how I was feeling I burst into tears. I was so embarrassed that I cancelled my next appointment and never went to see her again.

Late one night, talking with a friend I became pretty upset— anxious, more than anything. He asked me if I had loved the person who had hurt me. I said yes, and I remember feeling detached from the conversation, almost as though I was watching myself, and I thought, 'What are you talking about?' He held me and we were quiet. Then my sense of anxiety rose and suddenly I let out an ear-splitting scream. He held me, then stood by me and prayed while I shook, cried and shrieked. I think he thought I was possessed, and that the screams were evidence of the release of that. I was terrified. Even now, I don't know how to interpret that event.

A few days later my husband and I went away for a coastal weekend with the young people from our church. We hadn't seen most of these people for months, and I felt very distant from everyone. The emotional pain was like a rock in my chest. On the Saturday afternoon a friend asked me if I was OK and I fell apart. She walked with me on the beach, and I was hysterical. I remember saying to her through tears of despair, 'I prayed that it would stop and it didn't work!' I knew that this was related to my childhood, but I didn't know how, and again I felt as though I was not really there, as though I was watching myself. My friend was so helpful. She was prepared to reach in, walk with me, listen to me, hold me, and let me fall apart and cry. She asked how she could help me and I appreciated that; it was very respectful. She didn't need to say much—just her being there was enough.

Some weeks later I went to a weekend conference for women who had been sexually or ritually abused as children. I was scared to death, yet feeling almost like an imposter. In the stories and artwork of other women I heard and saw the feelings I couldn't articulate. I felt as though I had an affinity with these women; I just had no clear memories to prove to myself that I was right.

Eventually I went back into counselling, hoping that I could come to understand whether the experiences I remembered really were abuse, and to look at the problems in my life at present which I believe may be related to those experiences—difficulties with developing closeness to people and consequent loneliness; difficulties with trust and with sex and in my relationship with my husband; deep shame, guilt and depression. Now, I can say that I was molested by my father and that I am coming to believe that it wasn't my fault.

Just getting this far has taken me so long, and I feel there is still a long way to go, but I can look back and see progress. I believe that you need to be ready to talk, and you can't push that. Some days I feel that I am going forwards, some days I don't. I pray a lot. I find that not many people are willing or able to listen to my pain, and I find it hard to reach out to people. But along the way I have found that two people I knew before I started to deal with all this have also experienced abuse. We are able to share our difficulties with each other, and that helps.

Lynette Adams

◆

THE MYTH OF FALSE MEMORY

We find it shocking that there is a new label which attempts to discredit survivors, and behind which perpetrators can hide. Most people know very little about the issues faced by people who were abused as children, and the media are very one-sided in their approach, concentrating on the tiny percentage of false accusations rather than the hundreds of thousands of real memories. There is no mention of the fact that there are plenty of survivors who have been able to substantiate what they have remembered. The debate hinders our healing, scares therapists—our greatest allies—and makes it even more difficult for us to face our pain.

Survivors feel very strongly about the false memory myth. As well as being grossly unfair, it serves no purpose other than to slow down our healing. Our knowledge is based on our own experience. Those of us whose lives have been transformed by recovering our memories and healing from the events they restored to our consciousness know our truth far better than any professional who has not been through the experience.

It is incredibly hard to see the head of psychiatry at a leading Australian university declare on national television that there is no such thing as repressed memory of traumatic childhood events. Where does that leave me? What is happening to me if none of what I remember is true and my experience is not real? How can I have faith in myself and in what I'm experiencing when the 'experts' can't agree on the validity of what's happening to me?

Jan Watson

◆

The whole 'repressed memory' controversy has become so sensationalised and mystified as to be blown out of all proportion. The concept of repression is nothing new. I studied it when I did some basic psychology over 15 years ago. What we are witnessing now in the case of repressed memory therapy is the same insensitive handling of a subject that we saw—and still see—in the case of rape and incest over the last, say, ten years. People have a hard time accepting that such unpleasant things occur.

Do they not realise that their denial amounts to a further abuse of those who have already suffered? They obviously do not under-stand how hard it is, and how vital to the survivor, to summon up the courage to admit to themselves and their own circle of friends and family that something unspeakable happened to them—through no fault of their own.

Joan Burns

◆

I wonder how many people who read the reviews of *Stoker*, that recently released book about a survivor of Auschwitz who remem-bered his role at the camp forty years later, decided that he just 'remembered' it for the money? How many said that he couldn't possibly have forgotten it? How many claimed that important memories just can't be 'lost'? Funny that it's only when it's about childhood abuse that people get so insistent about what we do and don't forget.

Phillipa Brennan

◆

Initially the 'false memory' issue left me feeling sick and crazy. I avoided it like the plague, yet it became clear to me that if I wanted peace, I was going to have to address what it raised for me. I believe we face what we can in our own healing time, and it is difficult to come to terms with the reality of abuse in such a hostile climate. However, as survivors we can view the false memory myth as a challenge which can strengthen our healing.

For me it was a process of looking within and evaluating my five-year journey through the memories of a series of sadistic rapes by a family friend when I was aged between eight and ten. Did I make it up? Was I led into a false belief? The answer is an emphatic 'No!' Although I was in therapy at the time, these memories were certainly not 'suggested' or 'implanted'. They came about quite spontaneously as I sat alone one afternoon, wondering why I felt so strange. It is six years later now, and it's been a hard slog, but with my strength and the strength of those who love me, I am now a capable, confident woman who moves without shame.

Louise Plummer

When all the stuff about false memories came out a part of me was thankful that I hadn't blocked out everything—though most of the time I wish I hadn't remembered any of it.

Juley Taben

The false memory accusation has caused our family a great deal of pain and unwanted publicity. To turn on the television or pick up a newspaper and have my ex-husband stating that my daughter's memories are false is to me a cowardly way of dealing with her accusations of sexual abuse.

I believe Angela's memories to be totally her own and true, and I marvel at her strength in dealing not only with her memories of the abuse but also her father's way of shifting the blame.

Barbara Hodson, mother of Angela Forsberg

For years I have lived with a silent mind
    and a barrenness infused in my soul.
So when at last the dam broke, and the memories came
        forth,
    I assumed I would never be whole.

And the constant denial from the source of my pain
    and his heartless contempt for my fears,
So shattered my faith in the voice of that child
    who had known his cruel teachings for years.

For she never forgot the scars he had left,
  and when she finally found a voice
It hurt so much that the words that I spoke
  were assumed as a matter of choice.

Angela Forsberg

♦

People who recover memories of childhood sexual abuse. Who are they? Sufferers from 'false memory'? Neurotic, unhappy people, looking for someone to blame for their unsuccessful lives, finding compliant therapists and making money out of devastated and disbelieving parents?

So where does that leave me? At 28 I was pretty happy with myself and my life. I had married very young and had four children, and while the marriage had failed I was in the throes of rebuilding my life quite successfully. I adored my children and had a good relationship with them, and I had many good friends. I was young, pretty and attractive to men—more importantly, to men I liked. It was a pity that all these relationships seemed to hit some impenetrable barrier, but I thought this was just bad luck, and anyway I had time on my side. I was at university and doing very well. I was also one of those dreaded 1970s superwomen: managing very young children along with full-time study and part-time work. A friend once said to me, 'I don't understand you. At the end of the day my kids are driving me insane and I'm climbing the curtains. I can't wait for [my husband] to come home. But nothing ever fazes you.' And I thought it didn't.

But I did have a problem: I kept getting sick. Physically sick. Seriously sick. I began to have episodes when my speech would became slurred and I had trouble walking. I was diagnosed as epileptic, then as possibly having a brain tumour. These symptoms suddenly came to an end. A year later I developed uncontrollable bleeding, which became so bad that I needed a series of transfusions and finally, before I was 30, a hysterectomy. Then I started to have very long amnesic blackouts. I was scared witless.

I just wanted to find out what was wrong with me and then go back to my happy life. I went to three people. The first was a specialist physician, who said that I was in excellent physical condition though I seemed to have a difficult life, the second was an iridologist who said that he could not immediately tell me what was wrong but whatever it was, I was doing it to myself, and the third was a psychotherapist who said he believed he could help me.

And he did, but not until we had battled my absolute refusal to give any credence to anything I told him that suggested sexual abuse. While I raised images of nightmarish clarity, which I had always had, I fiercely insisted that they could not possibly lead to the conclusions that to him were obvious. Over a very long period I kept warning him against being deceived by me, agonising over whether I wanted to intrigue him or provide him with something 'juicy'. I could hear what I was saying, but I 'knew' it wasn't true. I wondered what in fact had happened to account for these images—I absolutely refused to grace them with the name of 'memories'—and I thought that one day I would find an explanation that would allow me to have back my own familiar world. He did not rush to provide any explanation. He did not tell me what had to be, and he did not tell me what could not be. He listened to me. He always said that no one could know the truth but me. But he was wrong. My mother could, and finally, after my father's death, she admitted the truth about what he had done to me.

Harriet Phillips

◆

I have three abused daughters whose abuser is often believed when he tells people that they are suffering from 'false memories'. If people could only see them in the pain and the hell of it all they would know that not only does one not wish to recall the horror, one would run a mile from it if one could.

My daughters have a very good but cagey psychologist—he can't be sure who might turn on him.

I think the 'false memory' campaign is so unfair to my daughters. If they cannot speak about the horrible abuse, how can they move forward in their lives? If someone who fought in Vietnam goes to a psychologist and says he has been having flashbacks of killings, etc., would the psychologist be so afraid of being sued that he'd be unable to ask: 'Were you in the war?'

F. Hayden

✦

I think we all need to thank the 'false memory' people. If it hadn't been for their nonsense I would never have gone public about my own abuse, and ASCA would never have started. We have to keep on reminding ourselves that we know our own truth. Fifteen years ago children who were admitted to hospital with broken bones as a result of parental violence were diagnosed as having 'brittle bones'. Truth always comes out in the end. It's just that the medical profession is sometimes a little bit slow!

Liz Mullinar

✦

I found Richard Guilliatt's articles in the *Sydney Morning Herald* very disturbing. I think that in the flood of publicity about 'false memory' the concerns of the survivors of child sexual abuse are not being considered. Of course the perpetrators will deny doing anything wrong, and being able to label the victim's memories as false is wonderful for them.

It is very common for victims of child sexual abuse to be so traumatised that the memory is successfully buried, sometimes for many years; this is how the child survives. This is how I survived.

Good counsellors do not implant ideas in their clients' minds; they assist them to retrieve their memories and deal with them. Survivors do not want these things to have happened, they are not gloating or happy about the memories, but eventually, once they have dealt with them, they will be able to live reasonably contented lives.

I appreciate that there is a difference between the victim being satisfied that what is remembered is true, and satisfying the requirements of the law. What concerns me is that the publicity given to the false memory myth creates more doubts and hassles for survivors, whose memories are far from false: the victims are blamed yet again, and the perpetrators are believed.

Jean McKendrick

◆

When I suffered the pain of sexual abuse as a child, it was so traumatic for me to understand how a protector and trusted one could actively hurt me that I blocked out all memory of it. I lived a troubled life (not consciously aware of the abuse, yet far from happy) for ten years. Then one day seven years ago, the first time I saw my current therapist, he simply asked me if I'd been sexually abused, and this prompted me to remember. There are many cynics who would claim that merely asking the question put 'false' memories in my mind, 'memories' of incidents that were a figment of my (or my therapist's) imagination.

Yet I find that very hard to believe. The last seven years have been very difficult for me. For nearly two years I was unable to work, simply being traumatised by the memories that kept bombarding me. My ensuing depression put me into a psychiatric hospital for about eight months in total, and during that time I tried to end my life three times by taking drug overdoses, and continued the self-abuse by slashing myself. It took me eight years to complete a three-year university degree, as I had to keep dropping out when I had breakdowns.

For a year after recovering my first memory, I felt too ashamed to tell anyone about it, even my closest friends. I felt I was to blame for the abuse, and couldn't even put the label 'abuse' on it. I found it very difficult to talk with my therapist about what had happened, and he never pushed me to do so, believing rather that I should take things in my own time. So why would I invent memories of abuse? Was my life really so boringly uneventful that I needed years of depression and suicidal tendencies to liven it up? Did I really want to cause a huge divide in my family through my allegations?

'Self-deception' is said to be one of the causes of 'false memory'. But why would those claiming to have been abused deceive ourselves into believing something that causes us feelings of guilt, depression, powerlessness, helplessness, shame, fear, pain, panic, self-loathing and great discomfort?

'Imagination' is another great one! When I confronted my abuser with the fact that he had orally raped me, he said, 'Maybe you sat at my feet and I asked you to put your head in my lap, and you imagined the rest'! What an imagination I must have had as an eight-year-old! To talk of having a penis in my mouth, when at eight I hadn't even been told what a penis was; to know the sensation of choking, gagging and feeling dizzy, when I had no comparable sexual experience outside the abuse.

Yet I take on board the accusations of 'false memory' even when those accusations are far from the truth. And accusations are what they are—putting victims into a position where they are seen as the ones at fault, rather than the perpetrators. I have my fair share of times when I think that I've made everything up, that surely this couldn't have happened to me, that my so-called abuser couldn't do those things, that I must have imagined it all. Yet I keep coming back to the knowledge that there is no reason for me to have made these things up. In a profit-loss ratio, I lose a lot more than I gain from the memories.

Survivors of child abuse have enough to deal with in facing the reality of their past without people accusing them of being the ones at fault—the ones destroying the lives of their perpetrators. When it comes down to it, no matter what strange sort of comfort we might gain from being the 'victim', we would rather have our lives back.

Mono

◆

I find the phrase 'recovered memories' very cumbersome. It is simplistic, and fails to explain the many processes involved when we go through and piece together a true historical narrative of our lives. Because of this it leaves people and what they are going through open to accusations of so-called 'false memory'. I think that we recall memories, aspects and facts about our lives that have been dormant. To talk of memories, true or false, is absurd and clinically simplistic. To me it is language created by lay people in a backlash of denial and refusal to accept the incredible incidence and prevalence of abuse, and in particular of incest and sexual abuse.

The media coverage has been the cause of many falls and stumbles in my therapy. I have been tougher on myself than any supporter of the false memory myth could ever have been. I have questioned over and over again the reliability of my thoughts and feelings because I am unable to 'prove' that the relationship with my father was incestuous.

The desire for me to have proof is not for me to believe myself, although that would make things easier, but for others who question me to see, to believe, and to know, to validate my experience and mirror my reality. Without this, I feel alone in my fight, despite the numerous people who support me.

Nobody saw what was happening to me. I know that at various times I tried to tell, but nobody listened to me. When nobody would validate me, reflect my reality, it turned into my unreality— and became buried deep within me.

Eva Gordon

◆

Each time I hear a person's story being discredited by so-called professionals who put it down to 'false memory', I feel angry that these victims are having to suffer further abuse. It is difficult enough already to hang on to our own truth, when denial is so much easier.

Elizabeth McMinn

✦

Some critics state with deliberate cynicism that memory appears to improve with therapy—a veiled suggestion of 'implantation'. I would respond: of course memory improves. Patients' defence mechanisms are gradually removed through therapy. As the defences come down, trust increases—and out comes the information.

It takes time for the truth to emerge because a violated, abused person has learned not to trust. It is painful. As children we experience our primary caregivers as gods. Imagine our sense of betrayal when we eventually realise their violation of us. We go into denial. We don't want it to be true, so we reject the memories and eventually repress them altogether.

Andrew Jacobs

✦

One thing has never been explained. Why would therapists bother to put memories into our heads? Would it cure us of our symptoms? No. Would it make us feel better? No. Would we continue to pay this therapist to heal us? No.

Only 5 per cent of survivors ever accuse their abuser. Most of us are happy just to heal ourselves, so why are we thought of as attention-seeking, mad people when we are attempting to heal?

Rodney Boxen

✦

We shall not cease from exploration
And the end of all our exploring
Will be to arrive where we started
And know the place for the first time.

T.S. Eliot, Little Gidding *(The Four Quartets)*

CHAPTER TWO

✦

How abuse affects us

'If a child is made fearful within itself, it holds back its true emotions. If we are not allowed to express our true self, the self we express becomes false. Fear, not hate, is the opposite of love. If we cannot feel or express love, we feel fear. We become afraid of life. Unable to love ourselves or even believe we are worth loving, we begin to doubt the very existence of love or happiness.'

Allegra Taylor, *Prostitutes*

Abuse of any kind has a profound effect on our development, our emotional growth, our health and our personality. We are all born looking for love, which is a human need as necessary for healthy growth as food and warmth. If we are mistreated in any way—neglected or harshly punished, constantly criticised, ridiculed, sexually or ritually abused, made to feel insignificant and unwanted—we will grow up feeling badly about ourselves.

We are brought up to believe that what adults tell us is true: apples are good for us, the sky is blue, we mustn't play with knives because they can cut us. Believing what we are told is the way we learn about the world we live in. So if an adult tells us that we are utterly stupid, that we must get out of their sight or they'll kill us, that touching our teacher's penis is good, that we are evil because we allow them to rape us, that we must never get angry or stand up for ourselves because it shows how bad we are and that we deserve to be hit before Mummy locks us in a room on our own for hours and hours—all this we will also believe.

And the result? We learn to suppress our feelings and to disconnect from events that might overwhelm us, even to the extent of splitting into different personalities. This necessary self-protection also prevents us from being able to feel really happy, and may lead to depression or to emotional pain so severe that suicide seems the only escape. If our abusers are people we look to for love, care, protection or guidance (which includes almost everyone a child is likely to know), their ill-treatment will make us believe that we are bad, unlovable, undeserving of care and respect. We grow up with low self-esteem and a lack of self-confidence. We may believe that everything that happens is our fault, and become filled with guilt and shame. We may learn that we will not be believed when we try to tell our dangerous or shameful secret. We discover that big and powerful people hurt people who are smaller and less powerful, so we feel afraid of being powerless and may turn into bullies, or feel so powerless that we are ourselves bullied. We learn that the world is an unsafe and painful place, and in order to protect ourselves and minimise the pain inflicted on us, we are likely to become either aggressive or submissive.

Above all, we are governed by fear rather than learning through love. A child who has grown up with fear finds it difficult to trust, difficult to believe that the world is a nurturing, exciting place to explore, and that living can be a great adventure. So much is stolen from us when fear becomes a constant companion.

There is almost no aspect of ourselves that abuse in childhood does not influence. We are likely to either become hard-driven perfectionists, constantly striving to achieve; or abandon the possibility of ever achieving anything because we believe we are hopeless. If we fear others and have learned to dislike ourselves, it is almost impossible to like other people and form close relationships with them—we may be condemned to a life of loneliness. The need to drown our fears can lead to addictions: drinking too much, taking drugs, overeating or being unable to eat are all signs of distress common among survivors. The tension of suppressed anger and outrage, of fear and depression, can lead to poor physical health: headaches, backache, digestive or respiratory problems, to name but a few everyday symptoms. The suppressed anger can be expressed inappropriately in acts of violence and destruction against the society which has allowed this to happen to us.

One way in which our physical and emotional difficulties will emerge is in our sexual relationships. This is particularly true for those who have suffered sexual abuse, though emotional and physical abuse also make us fearful of intimacy and of letting others touch us (or make us value ourselves so little that we do not protect ourselves from further abuse as adults). Although we were made to feel that our bodies are bad, they are not: it is our abusers who were at fault.

In this chapter, we have included a section on survivors' experiences as parents. Being a parent is never easy; for us it is even harder. How can we bring up our children confidently and lovingly when our own childhood experience was difficult and painful? One of the strongest motivations to heal comes from the realisation that however hard we try, our childhood will affect not only ourselves but also our children. Our recovery helps to break this intergenerational cycle.

It is comforting to discover that many of the personality traits we dislike in ourselves, the inadequacies that we give ourselves a hard time about, are common to all those of us whose childhood was damaging. Troubling feelings, ill-health, the sense of total inadequacy, attempts to mask the pain through addictions, fatigue and depression, are all normal responses to abnormal experiences. Understanding how much we have in common with other survivors can be an important first step towards challenging the negative messages about ourselves that we were given in childhood. As children, we had so little choice. As adults, we can choose to look at ourselves and our circumstances in new ways and change our behaviour.

It is inspiring to realise that if we learned to feel badly about ourselves, we can also learn to feel good about ourselves; if we learned to respond with fear to other people and unfamiliar situations, we can discover how to respond in new ways. All these negative feelings and responses to life were taught us; we were not born with them. This means we can also unlearn them. We can change, leave behind the parts of our personality that were forced on us, and discover our true selves. We can be lovable, affectionate, open, trusting. We do not need to cut off (dissociate) when anything threatens to become too emotional for us. Most important of all, we can rediscover how to feel our emotions fully; we can live in our bodies and not always in our minds.

OUR HEARTS, MINDS AND BODIES

When we first start acknowledging our pain it is incredibly difficult to separate what is the result of our abuse and what is not. We are often very anxious not to treat our abuse as an excuse for our feelings of inadequacy, our fears, our physical weaknesses, our outbursts of anger. We may struggle against these feelings, rather than realising that they were learned in response to what was happening to us. Anything that helped us to survive, that brought us to the point where it is safe enough to begin to face the truth, deserves to be honoured rather than despised, denied or rejected. There are no internal enemies—just wounded parts of ourselves still waiting for the love that was absent or betrayed in childhood. It is very validating and comforting to find we all share common traits, and armed with this knowledge it becomes easier to take an honest look at ourselves and try to move forward.

Many of the effects of my personality that I have been able to change I used to think were just negative personality traits. Triumphantly, they are not. My sense of worth was so diminished by my abuse that I became a traditional doormat. I always assumed I was just a wimp. I became an intensely fearful person. I could not understand why anybody would want to be friends with or love somebody as dirty or tainted as I believed myself to be. (But that was my abuser's definition, and is no longer mine!) One of the scariest things was always feeling different from others. Now I know I am indeed different, and I love and accept my differences.

I created a false self—I thought if I tried to be better I would be abused less. It didn't work, and I now know why. It is because abuse is not really about *you*, it is about those who hurt you. Nevertheless, throughout my teenage years I acted out the badness that I felt I was. By the time I was 12 I saw myself as just a lump of meat, good enough only for men's sexual needs. It blighted my perception to the extent that I was not able to see anything wrong with abuse towards myself. Other people, yes, but me, Louise, no. If someone raped or otherwise abused me I accepted that as my lot. I stayed in violent relationships. My whole view of myself reflected that of my abusers. Yet, wonderfully, I have learned that I do not have to share their view. How freeing this is!

Abuse can set up destructive patterns, and becoming aware of this is the first step in changing them.

Louise Plummer

◆

I don't know that I can get over the shame and guilt. My therapist repeatedly tells me that I didn't do anything wrong, but the nasty feelings still remain. I think I might die if anyone I work with or any of our acquaintances were to find out what happened to me. I wrestled for a long time with the idea that I was somehow making this up and that I might end up crazy like my crazy mother. Now I understand that this is the way these things work.

Rowena Robinson

◆

Many years ago as a baby I suffered abuse at the hands of a medical practitioner. It was truly a long time ago, as I am now retired. This abuse has been behind a lifelong anxiety condition, and it has taken an extraordinary effort on my part to deal with the symptoms.

I have been terrified of doctors for most of my life. At a tender age (less than two years old) I was taken to the surgery for treatment on my left arm, which I had broken the previous day. The break was a 'greenstick' fracture, and it had already begun to mend.

Without using any anaesthetic the doctor re-broke the arm before resetting it. I don't know who held me while the doctor worked on my arm, but I have been told that my uncle (who took me to the doctor) fainted. The experience was so traumatic and devastating that I have lived my life in fear ever since.

My school years were full of tension. I realised that if any measure of success was to come my way I had to have a 'cover-up' mechanism, and not reveal my real, fearful self. Despite my efforts, from time to time my anxiety would be so severe that I needed medical attention. The visits to doctors would be a trauma in themselves, with my blood pressure rising extremely high. Medication was the standard treatment, and on one occasion a doctor advised me to 'pull myself together'. Another time a medical specialist suggested that something in my past might be responsible, but doubted whether it was worth pursuing.

Later, with another doctor, I undertook relaxation therapy (medical hypnotherapy). This helped, but did not cure my malady. It was like pouring concrete over the problem: in time the concrete breaks up and the problem resurfaces.

Quite by chance I was referred to an understanding psychologist. From time to time since then I have had therapy to rid myself of the terror that has been a part of my life. I have made good progress, and I am happy to say that life has never been better.

Ron Hicks

◆

I had to learn as an adult to speak up for myself, because when I was a child I was taught not to, and became scared that people would trample all over me and try to disempower me whenever I tried to say what I thought or to defend myself. For a long time I allowed others to have power over me. I had to work hard to find my own voice and get my power back again.

Taylor Shane

◆

When I first started working with survivors and talking with them through ASCA, I found it difficult to understand why so many survivors had been abused more than once in their lives. Did they ask for it in some way? It was all made clear to me when I remembered my own second rape at the age of fourteen. It happened because as soon as I was attacked I went into 'victim mode': I felt powerless again, as I had been as a small child, and did not know how to stop what was happening. I was like a kangaroo held in the spotlight by a shooter. Until we recognise this victim mentality in ourselves and heal, sadly it can happen again and again.

Liz Mullinar

◆

I lost the ability to trust at a very early age, because to trust meant that I would be hurt. The one person I should have been able to trust was my father, and I couldn't. I should have been able to trust him to look after me, but he never did. He always had a hidden agenda. I was never able to trust my environment or my perceptions or my reactions or my own understanding of reality and its meaning. I felt that what happened was wrong, but as my father said otherwise I had to conclude that the fault in judgement was mine. So not only did I learn that I could not trust other people, I also learned that I should not trust myself. As an adult I have had to learn to trust myself all over again. Trust is essential to all relationships, and the lack of it has at some point harmed almost all my friendships.

I am still acutely distrustful and suspicious of men, especially those near my father's age. I fear them. If my own father hurt me, why shouldn't all other men also have that potential? My father should have nurtured me, protected me, and instilled trust and respect in me, but he did not. I dislike socialising with a lot of men, so I do not like the club or pub scene. I just cannot cope with it. I feel inadequate and incredibly ill at ease and frightened. When I try to confront this problem by going to a pub I feel intensely anxious and experience panic attacks, auditory hallucinations and depression. It all affects my life in so many ways.

My abuse makes me feel vulnerable and incredibly inferior to others. Because I find it terribly hard to trust, I avoid closeness with others so that I don't have to risk getting hurt again. This fear of getting hurt and of being rejected is deeply entrenched within me. I am angry not only at what my father did but also at his friend, who abused me too. Yet I find myself directing this anger—and with it, bitterness—at those closest to me, particularly any man with whom I become close. I resent my mother, who I feel knew (if only subconsciously) what was going on, but did nothing to protect her only daughter from two abusive men. Rather she always encouraged me to spend a great deal of time with my father, and referred to me as 'Daddy's little girl'.

Another legacy is the feeling of being unloved as their child, which is devastating and incredibly painful. What is more, my parents managed to create a family situation where I felt completely alone and isolated. I had no one to turn to for help, and thus suffered in silence for much longer than I should have.

Here are the ways the abuse affected me:
- psychosomatic symptoms, e.g. headache, stomach problems
- a great need for privacy
- depression and auditory hallucinations
- self-harm, e.g. cutting my wrists
- suicidal thoughts and actions
- an inability to stand up for myself and say no to things
- low self-worth and self-esteem
- little self-confidence
- guilt, humiliation, shame
- fear of being alone and in the dark

Penny Stevens

◆

I find it impossibly difficult to have someone in authority over me. I suppose it's because as a child I had no authority. I have to remind myself that there must be people in authority in this world, and they won't all abuse that position of power.

Liz Mullinar

◆

It's so hard to learn that it's OK to stand up for myself, that standing my ground won't always mean that I'm banished to my room or punished for 'answering back'. When I was a child even asking why I had to do something was completely unacceptable: unquestioning obedience was the only acceptable response to being told what to do. And as for expressing an opinion that differed from that of my parents and older siblings—unthinkable! I suppose it's not surprising that I still struggle against the feeling that anyone with authority has the right to overpower me, and that their view should prevail even when I think I have a valid alternative to offer.

Candida Hunt

◆

My fear of violence is constant. Every situation I am in feels as though it is potentially a violent one. I have always had a problem expressing opinions of any kind for fear of angering others. Anger is an emotion I only express inwardly, because I was never allowed to express it outwardly as a boy; it was only met with more anger and violence. I still feel as if everyone wants to hurt me.

I have a great deal of difficulty talking in a group in case I say anything that people will take offence at. In situations where discussion turns to argument I cannot speak for fear of anger. I do not talk even in normal situations for fear of being singled out or involved in a situation that may get out of my control. I need to be in control of my surroundings at all times.

These are the rules I learned to live by:

- Anger is violence
- If no one notices me I will be safe
- Keep to myself and avoid conflict
- I accept abuse, I do not have the power to defend myself
- Others must not like me, I do not know how to respond to affection
- I must always do everything right
- I'm afraid of getting into trouble
- I'm still the child I was
- I don't have anyone to look after me
- At work, socially or out shopping, I must do what others suggest so as not to get into trouble
- If I state my own opinion I am likely to be attacked.

I'm beginning to find qualities other than fear in myself: courage, determination, strength. No one else is giving me these things; I did not obtain them, they are a part of me. Mine is not the weakness, fear, uncontrolled aggression, sneakiness, perversion; they are what I was given. They are not mine. I can ask for help— this is strength!

John T.

◆

I sometimes want to punish myself. When I am really angry I pull at my toenails. Sometimes I see how long I can go without food. The longest I've managed so far is eleven days. I still drink lots, and take vitamin pills so my husband won't notice and so that I can still function.

Juley Taben

◆

When abuse is perpetrated by those who profess to love and care for us, those we depend on for our existence, the effects are devastating. Of course no one ever talks about it, because 'everyone knows that children lie'; children 'do not know what they are talking about' and 'cannot be trusted'. So we learn to split off, pretend to have a life where things are nice and loving and safe. We learn very early on to read signs, very subtle and conflicting clues. We learn how to 'disappear' when we have no control over what someone does to us that is hurtful or damaging. We grow 'tough'. We become very independent—while inside we seem never to grow up.

We may become very capable people as a result of all this. The difficulties arise when we begin to heal. We open up the dark corners, the hidden truths, the real memories instead of the ones we created to help us through our childhoods. That is when we fall apart, have to find the broken pieces, and try—usually with a lot of help—to put together a person from the fragments of personality that resulted from our experiences. It can be done; a lot of us have begun to do it. And though it is a very painful process, it is very satisfying.

Peter Sandford

✦

I have spent 30 years hiding from my feelings. I have never known what love might really feel like. Even now, if I feel like loving someone it is still mixed up with fear. The feeling of being an outsider, always on the outside looking in, is still there: feeling that there was something wrong with me, but not knowing what; doing things that ultimately would be self-destructive. I would get to the verge of success in work, and then throw it all away as I could not cope with the success. I had no self-esteem or self-confidence. I was unable to believe that I was a good, caring, worthwhile individual, or to accept compliments—it was easier to accept putdowns and abuse than to believe anything positive about myself. I was unable to cope with anyone being aggressive towards me.

Stuart Andrew Robertson

✦

The effects of the abuse were many while I was growing up. I knew I was different, I knew I was bad, I knew I was unacceptable, and I knew what was happening was wrong, though I didn't dare tell anyone about it. I could never get really close to anyone, never had a best friend as I couldn't share my closest secret, my darkest fears, or let my guard down. It's hard to be eight years old, sitting in class and worried that you are pregnant.

Carmol Morley

◆

We grow up with a marked lack of self-esteem, a conviction that we are unworthy or 'dirty' in some way, and most damaging of all, we believe in our victimisation.

These beliefs ensure that we then attract to ourselves an endless succession of situations that reinforce or play out the circumstances of our early childhood. As time goes by the belief that we are victims becomes more and more entrenched until it is an integral part of our lives. When I first went to a kinesiologist with three specific ailments, he traced them all back not only to sexual abuse but also to my subconscious belief that I am—inescapably—a victim.

Learning to understand the effects of my abuse has answered the following questions:

- Why I became addicted to drugs
- Why I had a victim mentality ('It's not fair', or 'Why me?')
- Why I enjoyed courtship rituals, but the moment sex appeared in a relationship I freaked into anxiety and fear, and was in pain during intercourse
- Why I never had a satisfactory sexual relationship
- Why I never spent the night in the arms of the man I loved. One or other of us always went to our respective homes (just as my father and I had gone to our respective rooms)
- Why I had no sex at all between the ages of 35 and 60
- Why I had so many nervous breakdowns

- Why I endured forty years of psychosomatic pains
- Why I feared authority figures
- Why I went to pieces when faced with confrontation of any kind
  And much more ...

Margaret Wood

◆

We are very good at defending others, we just have to learn to treat ourselves as we treat other people.

Eloise Kaitlin

◆

When I was a child, humour was used sarcastically or to cover up feelings—not to express genuine amusement. My childhood led to my developing a personality that was morose, withdrawn, introverted, pessimistic and fearful. I grew up feeling that nothing I do is good enough, with a lurking fear of abandonment, with constant negative conditioning, unable to believe that any compliments paid to me are genuine, with no confidence in my abilities and with the 'subliminal tapes' of my parents' critical voices constantly replaying in my head.

I don't open up easily to people. I'm neither friendly nor outgoing, and still feel shy and socially inept. I often can't believe that anyone would find anything I say interesting or worthwhile.

When I recognised that I was growing into a carbon copy of my parents, I set about working to try and change my personality: trying to be sociable, unselfish, and to have lots of interests outside the home. Then I realised that I was trying to wear a glove that would never fit me. So I worked to make the glove I already had fit: to stop hating myself and to take advantage of my good points. It's not a crime to be introspective, quiet, and not to trust everyone on sight. Like everything else, these can be turned into good or bad things. If it had been left to my parents, I'd be conservative, frightened of my own shadow, dependent and selfish. But I'm not!

Jacqueline Frajer

◆

Sports captain, school captain, dux of the primary school. Trying to be the best. Trying to make up. Channelling my energy. Focusing on anything but the unresolved hell of what happened.

No close friendships because they might see what a bad child I really am. Playing the game. Trying to appear normal.

Spending many hours pretending not to be me. Fantasising about death: it is to be my crowning achievement.

Never good enough. The anger rages. The distraction of perfection is just that. And the anger rages.

Hannah Gunn

◆

The effects of the abuse are all-pervasive.
- Problems as a teacher: In my first two years of teaching I was unable to discipline the children because of my father's past domination of me and his heavy-handed physical punishments.
- The pleasure-pain issue: If something is good there must be something bad about it. Is it really all right for me to have a kitten, just for me to enjoy? She's female, so she can have kittens of her own. Incredible healing came through Pippi, and she still gives me so much pleasure.
- Physical touch: I constantly yearned for hugs and other signs of love and acceptance, yet gave negative vibes to others to stay clear.
- Submission: Total submission to those in authority was the result of obeying the Fourth Commandment, to honour one's parents. I found it impossible to say no to my father; it was a long time

before I realised that I was like a rag doll in relation to him.
- The need to be heard: I constantly sought someone who might listen to me, understand me, and help me resolve my pain.
- My opinion doesn't count: It was always ignored or quelled with threats. Only recently have I started to feel that I have something to say that might be worthwhile.

Julie Waddy

✦

I am 55 now, and as a consequence of childhood abuse I am more aware than ever of the sense of powerlessness that permeated my journey through life—and still pulls me up short on occasions. Suddenly I will become aware of tiredness, sickness, confusion and uncertainty, and then the penny drops. I am feeling powerless! And then I realise that I can take back my power, because to be human is to have been given power, and I let go of my fears and am able to act again as an adult.

Barbara Lumley

✦

ANGER
Slowly, precisely she slices at her skin with a knife.
Etching the cross. To protect her from Evil. From him.

Seeking divine intervention, though any intervention will
do. The blood attracts and repulses her. Bleeding.
She always seems to be bleeding.

But the cross cannot protect her from herself. It cannot
save her from the insatiable desire to hurt herself.
The recurrent theme that will become her life.

And the anger rages through her body. Anger at God and
anger with all of them for allowing this to happen to her.

It merges with the pain and transposes itself, becoming a chrysalis.

A chrysalis of self-loathing, self-hatred and despair.
The self-destructive, empty child awaits adolescence.
To be born again.
To be able to wage war against herself.
The sacrifice.

Hannah Gunn

◆

I am filled with an all-consuming anger about what my mother did to me. I'm angry that no one heard me when I was a child, angry that no one believes me now I am an adult. Because of my anger I became a professional soldier, because of my anger I took drugs to try and find peace, because of my anger I committed crimes and spent twelve years in jail. I have worked for two years to cure my drug addiction. My life has been destroyed by my mother—how do I cure my anger?

John Phillips

◆

I believe I have a better and wider understanding of personal pain because I've been through it, and I know what it is like.

Christine Gale

◆

Sobbing, I hold my dog as she dies.
She is gone now.
I hold her warm body tighter,
softly moaning and crying.
The floodgates have opened.

Her soft black fur becomes
the soft black hair of my sister.
Sorrow and intense pain
course through my body,
a medley of confusion and loss.

Emotional hiatus,
the precursor for feelings
locked away for a lifetime.
Suffering, sadness and distortion fuse
into oneness
and I am lost.

I weep for those I have lost.
I grieve
for what I had
stolen from me.
My sister, my mother, my childhood.
I weep for my distorted perceptions of life.

I mourn
the corruption of my capacity to love,
the exploitation of innocence
and my shame
for who and what
I am.

He insidiously ravaged
the soul of the child
and she learned
to hate herself.
She grew to know fear
and learned not to trust.
The child was deprived of dignity

and her right to choose
was pilfered.

I hold the warm body
of my dead dog,
and the burden of guilt and grief
is overwhelming.
My soul wails for
retribution.

Hannah Gunn

◆

I was disconnected from my body for so long that I was out of touch with everything. I lived my life in a daze, a fog, as I could not appreciate all the good things I had in my life. I feel like I have been only half alive, like a walking zombie—functioning, but that was all. I still have days when I am down, and feel: what's the use, is it really worth trying? There are other days when I feel OK. The biggest thing is learning to like my body and get in touch with it and with my feelings.

Linda Honey

◆

I was nine years old when the sexual abuse began, and 15 when it stopped. The oral sex was the worst thing that happened. I remember pleading for it not to happen, how I could not breathe, how my heart pounded, the panic when I thought he was choking me to death. I never forgot.

The abuse ruined my health. I was constantly sick, and unable to swallow my food. I was afraid of my strict, Victorian, domineering mother, who just yelled at me when I told her I could not swallow, and refused to let me leave the dinner table until my plate was clean. Sometimes I would sit there for two hours. This ritual was repeated day and night for years, and as the abuse continued I became sicker and sicker until eventually I lived on clear liquids. I was a living skeleton.

I felt I was in a hell from which there was no escape. I became so frightened of people that I would withdraw into my own little world. I was carrying this unbearable burden, and I felt my shoulders were not strong enough; I hated myself for being so weak. My mother always demanded perfection from me, and I felt I failed her; she later said I had been gutless as a child. I so much wanted her to love and hold me, and to hear her tell me that she loved me; but it was not to be. I hated my childhood.

I am now 55 years old, and I still suffer every day. It never goes away. Over the years I have had to cope with dry-retching, vomiting, chronic insomnia, nervous dyspepsia, irritable colon, migraines, chronic depression, panic attacks, fearful obsessions and guilt.

I know that I was not guilty. It was not my fault. It was my mother's: she put me in the care of my uncle, who lived just over the road so contact with him was constant, though she knew he had a bad reputation. When I pray I ask for God's help to forgive her; I'm trying.

I am still having difficulty in swallowing, but I can manage soft foods now. My swallowing worsens when I have to try to eat food in front of other people. I become quite ill—my mouth dries, my stomach hurts, and all appetite disappears. I panic. I have never lost my fear of choking to death. My psychiatrist tells me that all my symptoms are a result of my upbringing.

Children are so precious, such beautiful little human beings. They should be heard. Does anyone take the time to hear them?

Gay Darcy

◆

My experience left me with a legacy of inappropriate responses
and severe body memories. It was not uncommon for me to
shiver and shake, have nausea, headaches and diarrhoea when
I felt unsafe. I subliminally relived the abuse and the pain in
all my relationships, and set myself up to be victimised: like
the child of three, I was defenceless. Severe body memories
would inflict me when I was in a group—at business meetings,
parties and other social gatherings. These times (which might
have given me the means for healing and interaction) became
times of torment as I distanced myself from others in order to
cope. I also had times of regression, when I felt my size change
and my balance was affected. I would feel incredibly heavy, and
I didn't know how to write. Yet despite all this, on the surface
I generally appeared to be well-adjusted. I had made the mask
and had learned to wear it well, so well that the acceptance I
sought from others was not of me as I truly was, but of the
mask.

Joseph Elias

◆

All my life I suffered from frequent sore throats, laryngitis and
other respiratory problems. Since I have remembered the hand
around my throat that stifled my cries, nearly throttling me while
my life was threatened, and have healed from the memory, I only
rarely get throat infections or lose my voice.

Lily Pike

◆

I have experienced the physical effects of abuse in a way that is
like the slowing down of my whole system. That's what depression
feels like in my body. Anger, on the other hand, tends to speed
things up, resulting in blurred vision, palpitations and nausea, a
coldness sets in that requires more than a cardigan, and I constantly
want to wee.

I'm sure many other survivors will understand the physical effects of our histories in terms of sleeping. On the nights I couldn't sleep because every time I closed my eyes I saw 'him', I was ragged all the next day and half asleep in evening lectures.

Painful sexual intercourse at times when abuse memories have been playing havoc has also been a problem. Pains in the body parts that correspond with acts of abuse were also terrifying. This also happens with physical abuse that I've always remembered. When I wrote for the first time about my mother battering me, I began to feel all the fear of the eight-year-old girl, and had stomach pains where she used to kick me. As a child I used to be able to numb it so that it didn't hurt, a survival skill I later took into other abusive relationships. As the remembering adult, however, I felt the pain all over again.

Besides the anxiety, I think one of the worst things about the physical effects of my abuse has been the terrible lethargy I've experienced. For a time it was difficult for me to speak of my abuse because I would literally start to nod off. When I was being abused as a youngster I would feel this terrible, thick torpor over-take me. Protection, for sure, but a pain in the bum when one is trying to work with the issues. I had to wait until I was ready not to need the torpor any more.

As survivors, I believe it is healing to treat our bodies as impor-tant, and to be gentle. Although I still abuse mine with nicotine, and the fairly regular hangovers have yet to be resolved, I like to keep my body warm, sweet-smelling clean, and to walk for 40 minutes a day. It's a way of giving my body the respect my abusers never gave me.

Louise Plummer

◆

Through my teenage years I was first anorexic and then bulimic. I have an obsessive-compulsive disorder, and I have been treated for these symptoms for years. What my body was really crying out for was for me to deal with my childhood.

Diana Passoni

◆

When your gut tells you to run but you know you can't run fast enough or far enough to escape, it's the muscles at the front of your thighs that keep you upright where you are standing. They were the first part of my body to remind me of my pain. Much more was to follow.

I was diagnosed as needing surgery on both hands for carpal tunnel syndrome. I'm glad I didn't go through with the operation. The pains, the tingling, numbness and tension moved up to my elbows (diagnosis: tennis elbow), and then to my shoulders (diagnosis: RSI—repetitive strain injury). I developed walnut-sized lumps on my back and shoulders, muscle spasms, and increasingly violent headaches so severe that I would even black out for a few seconds. Scary stuff.

Physiotherapists told me that I had bad posture, and should stand up straight. My posture reflected the state of fear I walked around in—I had been whipped every day. I had also had to live with the emotional pain of never knowing if what I was saying or doing would be right or wrong, and what level of punishment would be meted out to me. Even when I was unwell and couldn't go to school, I was still not safe. My mother said my illness and asthma were psychosomatic—and according to her, this meant that I wasn't really sick, I just thought I was.

Years of lying tense in bed, waiting, feeling cold. Years of terror, not knowing whether I'm being spied on, whether I'm doing or saying something right or wrong, whether I will finally get it right now and gain approval. I was the human equivalent of a cringing dog with its tail between its legs, crawling on its belly.

I'm learning now about the pains in my body, and that although tracing them to specific causes won't fix them it will help me understand them: our physical bodies do reflect our emotional selves.

Linley Valente

✦

TEARS
Tears, tears, tears
Tears of emptiness
Tears of despair
Tears of loneliness
Tears of no one being there.
Tears of shame
Tears of denial
Tears of never knowing why.
Tears of anger
Tears of revenge—it won't be over even when it ends.
Tears of frustration
Tears of terror
Tears of self-harming
Tears of goodbye
Tears of suicide.
Tears on my pillow
Tears fill my bed
They just keep tumbling, there's no relief ahead.
Tears of sorrow
Tears of darkness
Tears of pain
Tears of grief
Tears that are torn from the soul—the soul that will never
    heal.
I am sad
Sad is me.
Will I ever again feel tears of happiness
Tears of joy

Tears of recovery
Tears of life
Tears of peace
Tears of contentment
Tears of love
Tears that I'm happy to be a part of life?
Cry, cry forever to clear away the pain,
Cry little girl, cry—you carry another's shame.

Carmol Morley

◆

MULTIPLE PERSONALITIES

Dissociation—cutting off from unpleasant events, refusing to think about difficult situations, denying feelings of discomfort or pain—is a normal human response. Everyone does it. The more traumatic the experience, the stronger this mental splitting is likely to be. It can be life-saving protection. Survivors understand this all too well. Distancing ourselves from the events that brought us such pain was the only way we could blot it out. Everyone also talks and argues with themselves: a responsible, 'adult' part may insist that we finish a piece of work while a 'child' part tugs at us to go out for a walk because the sun has just come out, or clamours for a piece of chocolate only to be admonished by a 'parent' part reminding that too much chocolate isn't good for us, or that we don't deserve a treat. Generally, we are aware of all the parts that make up the whole person we are.

If we are repeatedly exposed as children to unbearable experiences we may split off awareness completely to other parts of ourselves, particularly if there are repeated traumatic events and abuse. These other parts may then take on different roles—there may be an 'angry one', a 'protector', a 'victim'; any role the person cannot deal with—and develop into distinct personalities. The medical profession call this multiple personality disorder (MPD) and/or dissociative identity disorder (DID). We have chosen to use the term MPD, which is the one more often used by our contributors.

Multiple personality disorder usually develops before the age of six and is a response to bizarre and sadistic abuse. When a child feels completely overwhelmed and fears that it will die, and this situation is repeated again and again, the child's only defence is to disappear—to become someone else.

Some perpetrators, especially those who are involved in ritual or organised sadistic abuse, know about the child's ability to develop multiple personalities as a response to severe trauma and use it to their own advantage. They sometimes train different personalities to take on certain functions or jobs, 'jobs' which would be completely unacceptable to the 'host' personality, which is the part of the person who leads most of the daily life. These unacceptable 'jobs' can include staying in contact with the perpetrators and being sexually available to them.

A person who has developed multiple personalities may also perceive changes in body image: when they look in the mirror they see themselves as having differently coloured hair, or looking younger or older than they are. It is not unusual for such people to feel as if they are standing behind or looking down at themselves, watching what is happening but having no control over it. Some multiples have periods of amnesia or time loss. They might find themselves in places with no recollection of how they got there, or talking to people they don't recall having met before. It is not uncommon to find among their belongings clothes or other items that they cannot remember having bought. Friends may refer to shared events the multiple has no memory of attending. They may also find themselves writing in distinctly different handwriting over a period of time.

Dissociation, and even the development of multiple personalities, was once a life-saving reaction to an unbearable situation when there was no other way to escape the trauma. Later in life this defensive response to stress can prevent you from using your adult strengths and skills to protect yourself and take charge of your own life. You need to remember that when you were a child you did the best you could to protect yourself from emotional annihilation, and you must be proud of the fact that you survived.

In many ways it's a miracle that I'm alive to write this. My abuse started early, and lasted a long time. It was more than any one person could take, particularly a little child. So in order to cope, my mind played a curious and clever trick—it split.

The splits began in small ways. When I was being abused I simply let my conscious self fade into the background, and allowed some other part of me to take over. It was easy. I would stare at the blinds, drop my breathing down to a whisper and wander away from my body as though it was an uncomfortable suit I didn't like wearing. When the abuse stopped, I would come back into my body as a stranger; bewildered, hurt and relieved that it was all over for the moment. I don't think I really understood that I had been abused. If I had known the whole truth, I would probably have gone mad, so I didn't let myself. The parts of me that took over during the abuse kept their secrets well. 'I' was safe, and could get on with life as though nothing had happened.

But something *had* happened. The parts of my personality were growing in different directions. Some were coping with the abuse; others were going to school or playing with friends; still others were watching TV with the family or eating sardine sandwiches or hiding in corners of my mind in various states of shock. I was no longer one person. I couldn't be one person and survive.

I was confused and bewildered, never knowing which way to turn. It was as though I was being ordered to go in every direction at once, and each opposing order was so definite and compelling that I often found myself unable to move at all.

It was not until my early thirties, when I was diagnosed [with MPD], that the confusion turned into understanding. I was being ordered to go in different directions. The personalities who had suffered the abuse were telling me to hide at all costs; the healthier, more gregarious personalities were telling me to get on with my life. The different parts of me had long ago ceased to be simply parts of a whole; they had developed into distinct personalities in their own right.

Being multiple is never easy. There are difficult experiences to work through; there is a constant need to negotiate and compromise over who has control over our body and so gets to do what they want to do while the others must wait; exhaustion and self-mutilation and suicidal feelings have to be overcome.

But being multiple is never lonely, either. We give each other trouble, but we also help each other. Having been strangers for most of our lives, we are learning to work together and share this body in ways that give everyone a chance to learn or play or grieve or do whatever is necessary for them to become whole and healthy. It's an unusual life, but it is a life and, thanks to our own persistence and the help of our outside friends, we are still around to talk about it.

Amos

◆

Being a multiple is sometimes like riding a rollercoaster. When coming out of a dip there's no certainty who's going to be at the front and what's going to get said. It's living with a magnified despair that can depart as suddenly as it arrived: the door revolves and the mood changes. MPD is being in a shop, staring at an item while other voices and wills clash, wanting other foods, colours, whatever.

Despite the difficulties, there are many funny and lovely moments being multiple, and we have some happy and supportive times with other multiples. But being multiple is not a lifestyle. The others of us are not an 'inner child'. MPD is a disability.

Alison Stowe

◆

My children always remember what happened and never deny it, even when they seem to be 'someone else'. It is embarrassing when Robert is out somewhere, or we have a visitor, and suddenly he changes from an eight-year-old to a two-year-old, taking out his toddler's toys and regressing in his speech. But neither of them is as seriously affected as some people.

Lorelle Somerville, mother of Sarah and Robert

✦

'. . . Multiple personality
is more accurately described
as Dissociative Disorder . . .'

Yeah
that must be me
because I do dissociate
myself from the world
in a very dis-orderly way
because I've often
got to do it in a great hurry
a rush of panic
& bewilderment
& I kick up a lot of dust
when I struggle
& bump into things
when I run
& with my mind gone blank
& body moving
out of my control

yeah
dis-ordered dissociation

& the voices

in my head
argue
or all speak at once
all want their say
& that does get
very dis-orderly
& I call out
'Order! Order!'
& everyone
yells back their orders
for pies & coke
& fish & chips.

Lori Rickard

◆

DEPRESSION AND SUICIDE

You may have turned to this section in one of those moments of extreme despair—when life seems to be reaching a climax of unbearable pain. Sometimes even the relaxing bath, the teddy bear, writing out your feelings, talking on the phone, listening to 'the band that understands', or whatever else just isn't enough, and the damburst of painful emotions brings a flash flood. These are the times you don't think you can ever get through, and when you do, you're not sure how you did. What we (understandably) lose sight of is that each of these experiences can help to clear up the clogged streams, just like real rain.

Depression and suicidal feelings are almost inevitable effects of childhood abuse. Like dissociation, depression can be protective, a way of unconsciously avoiding feeling painful emotions that we fear will overwhelm us. But the price we pay for this protection is high. Depression isolates us, makes us feel unreachably alone, is a place of darkness where no light can break through. Sometimes the numb feeling of depression has another protective function: it makes us too exhausted and inert to harm ourselves.

Suicidal feelings are especially likely to arise when we are deep in our pain, when we are not yet able to confront it, to see that we are more than the pain, and begin to move through it. Suicidal feelings should not be viewed as an abnormality. They are not caused by 'less than adequate social interactions', 'negative thinking', 'simply being depressed' or 'a chemical imbalance in the brain', as people sometimes say to lessen their discomfort with such an extreme response to a life that has become unendurable. Feeling so desperate that we consider ending our life in order to put an end to our pain is a tragic, but normal response to the agony many survivors endure. We need to acknowledge the reality of this despair without being frightened of it, to help each other hear the feelings and the truth that lie behind the desire to die, and accept them.

At times the feelings and emotions are so strong, so huge, so engulfing. Suicide, self-harm and at times homicide are options that flit through my mind. It's the wanting to escape, the need for the pain to ease and the anger to quieten down that makes these options desirable.

Carmol Morley

◆

This is some of what I have learned about depression.
- Depression is . . . loneliness. A need to communicate your fear, grief and guilt (self-anger) at being lonely, without being abused for doing so.
- Depression is . . . physical symptoms similar to those of chronic fatigue syndrome: fatigue, joint pains, muscle cramps, headaches, burning pains, tingling, fungal infections, cystitis and skin rashes.
- Depression is . . . a situation that links back through layer after layer of comparable emotions to the earliest one in childhood. Thus fear becomes panic, grief becomes despair, anger becomes rage, guilt becomes overwhelming. Unless all the layers are dealt

with until the original one surfaces, depression will inevitably return again and again.

• Depression is ... panic attacks. Total abandonment. Nobody in the whole world is there for me. A feeling of being powerless, helpless and unable to cope.

• Depression is ... the fear of communicating our pain because it would exacerbate other people's pain, and cause them to hit out in self-defence or reject us in some way. So we repress our strongest need: love.

• Depression is ... loss. The loss of a home, a job, and above all of loved ones, especially when the loss links back to a childhood loss—a parting, an abandonment or an experience of rejection.

And these are some of my thoughts about suicidal feelings, which seem to be an almost inevitable result of depression if we don't get help early enough.

• Suicide is ... feeling unloved, unwanted and rejected.

• Suicide is ... fear of being unable to cope.

• Suicide is ... fear of being a personal failure, despite evident success.

• Suicide is ... deep lack of self-esteem.

• Suicide is ... fear of insanity.

• Suicide is ... feeling trapped in a situation that you can't get out of, that you hate and fear, and that you feel unable to cope with.

• Suicide is ... helplessness.

Margaret Wood

✦

Why am I writing this on suicide? Shouldn't I be dead? No, the living can also write about it, and I am one of them, writing from my own experience.

Why have I wanted to kill myself at all? Well, that is simple—*to end the pain!*

As a child I was badly hurt by my parents. Instead of giving life to me they in fact took life away from me. I have nothing to show for my existence but years of pain. I existed in the realm of abuse by them. As a child I was not loved, protected, nurtured or kept safe.

My whole life has been overwhelmed by fear, lack of confidence or belief in myself, low self-worth, feeling stupid and inadequate—just full of pain and suffering. Which is one hell of an existence, if you ask me.

Oh the pain—the pain is so great—I hate it! I have felt envious of those who have at least found peace in the final step . . . success in suicide. I'm here to share the pain with others who have felt as bad as this—you are not alone.

Suicide always strikes me as the answer, the solution, when all else seems to fail. To love yourself is the key, they say. It's bloody hard to do that when you have never been loved—especially by the most vital people in a child's life, your parents.

I died a long time ago—I've really been the walking dead. So killing myself would not be taking away my life . . . When is all this going to end for me? Is death the only solution?

I don't really trust what I am about to say. It's this—that I may have finally turned the corner in my pain. Thanks to a couple of contacts I have made recently, I may have finally found the key. I can even say, cautiously, that I've been feeling the best I have felt for a long time. Even the strong thought of suicide has subsided greatly.

I deserve that—don't I? To experience some light instead of darkness. To go beyond my 39 years. If I get to my 40th, I would hope that the next 40 years will be better. Life is still scary for me today—it's a constant struggle.

Suicide should not be the answer for anybody—but I sure understand it. The depth of pain is just incredible. People should not sit in judgement. My thoughts, care and understanding go out to those in deep pain and despair. My tears are there for you and me at this moment. Hang in there with me—let's walk the journey together.

Let our voices and pain be heard—let's help break the cycle and silence of abuse. Stay alive: if we are dead we will no longer be heard.

Janice Atkinson

◆

IF I CHOOSE
If I choose to die, would you see this deed
as you've seen my life: just a waste of time,
or regret your choice not to intercede,
as events brought change to your paradigm?

Would the deep relief from the pain I feel
be the sign you need to review with blame?
Would your knee-jerk acts let your world reveal
that behind our masks we are all the same?

Would you think that I should have worked things out?
Would you say nice things, in resentful tones?
Would you search for ways to displace your doubt,
before fear was linked to my silent bones?

Would you paint your world in a lighter shade,
as my life form changed to a memory?
Would the store-bought warmth of the bed you've made
hold back tears, which all but the blind could see?

Would your photographs of my haunting face
just be cast aside, as my frame was burned?
Would you think the world was a better place,
when the days had dragged till the calm returned?

If I choose to die, would a hindsight clue
cause regret for time that you would not take?
Would your son, at last, be a part of you,
or would

      I remain

           just a big mistake?

Brian Bell

◆

How many times did I think about suicide? It would be easier to count how many times I didn't.

Why didn't I do it? Well, I had children, and they had no one but me. But that works just so far and no farther. At a certain point I would think, 'But no one can expect me to go on suffering this much just because they need me'. It felt like just the latest example of how my role in life was limited to what others needed from me.

But what do we mean when we say 'suffering this much'? Suffering what? How? It is so much easier to understand physical suffering. I don't mean easier to endure, but easier to understand. We can all understand the terrible pain that drugs will no longer dull. What is mental suffering?

We often read that some people are 'just' depressed—as if that is somehow not as substantial as 'real' suffering. What was I suffering?

Isolation, above everything else. Not aloneness: I worked with a lot of people I loved, I had friends around me. But I couldn't reach anyone. I felt as if I were in a glass silo. I could see and appear to be in the world, but I couldn't touch it and no one could touch me.

The nuns had told me that hell wasn't really flames, and devils with tails and pitchforks. It was eternally being denied the face of

God, knowing for all time that you would be cut off from the source of love. I believed them. Of course I did, I already lived in hell. I didn't know how I had got there. I didn't really care about that. What I did care about was that I didn't know how to get out.

I must have thought about suicide thousands of times over the years, and always fought it off. Like an alcoholic, I will go just another day, always reserving the right, if it finally got too much, to give in and kill myself. I would not agree to stay alive only to be tortured.

And then I reached 'too much'.

I had managed to stay ahead till my children grew up and left home. I no longer owed myself to anyone. I knew they would grieve and I deeply felt that, but it was not enough to make me keep enduring.

I was very careful. I had a bottle of sleeping pills. I knew that you had to be sure not to vomit them up, and I knew that alcohol would 'make assurance doubly sure'. I had a shower; I washed my hair; I put on a clean nightie. I had bought a bottle of Scotch, and very slowly, very carefully I sipped the whisky and swallowed the tablets. Fastidious, competent, methodical—I was being myself to the last.

I had arranged for a friend to visit me the next day. I was determined that none of my children would find me (I was less caring of that unfortunate friend!), and I had left my front door unlocked. Just in case anyone called in and ruined everything by discovering me and making a rescue bid, I hid the bottle and all evidence of what I had done. If anyone came in (and no one was due to) I would look as if I had been drinking and had fallen asleep. No one would disturb me.

And the next morning I woke at my normal time.

I felt as if the ship had sailed and I was not on it. I couldn't understand. I was shattered. I felt as if I had gone 14 rounds with Muhammad Ali. My eyes felt as if they had been punched out, I was spaced out. And I looked perfectly normal. It was just the way it had always been. I had been to the edge of death, and no one could see a thing.

My brother-in-law rang during the day. He asked how I had enjoyed the Quantum programme the night before. I'd been watching it as I drank, and we discussed it. I said nothing about what had happened. After I got off the phone I thought, 'You're supposed to love him. You say you're close. You've just tried to kill yourself and you can't tell him. Reach out. It's your last chance.'

What had happened? I don't know. I didn't think it possible that I could be alive. I could only believe that God had intervened directly. I did not thank him for it. Where had he ever been when I needed him, and now he butted in. But I thought that he also seemed to be suggesting that it was worth keeping going, that there was something better for me than I had experienced so far. I couldn't believe that he had kept me alive only so I could live in misery. I agreed, unwillingly, to keep going. But I continued to reserve the right to change my mind, and next time to be absolutely sure I got it right. That was six years ago. I'm still battling. I haven't won yet, and sometimes I still regret missing my 'flight'. But I'm hanging in there.

Phillipa Brennan

◆

The torture and hurt inflicted on me between the ages of three and 22 has had a great effect on me. I am only 26 now, and so have been tortured for most of my life. I cannot shut this hurt off even though I have tried to. It is a part of me and it makes me who I am. It cannot be ignored. I deal with the sadness better than I used to. When I was younger I could cry for days and days and could never see any hope for my future. How could life possibly have something good to offer when all I had known was grief? I still get sad, I still cry and I still withdraw, but I am slowly realising that I can live with it and cope with this sadness.

The sadness has reached great depths. I have twice taken an overdose, and at the time I honestly believed that I could not go on any more. What really hurt was that I took the first one while I was still at school and living at home with my mother. I slept all weekend; no one noticed and no one seemed to care.

Penny Stevens

◆

I've never attempted it, but I have felt chronically suicidal during the last 19 years. Currently I'm free of it. One of my big fears is criticism and the accusation of 'self-pity'. I already felt so bad about myself, so unacceptable; what I desperately longed for was acceptance and care.

I don't know what to say about it. It's just been a big part of my landscape. The closest I got to doing it was at 27, when drunk and miserable. I'd been sexual with my counsellor and had just scored a job as a prostitute.

I angrily slashed my legs with a razor, and then held it to my wrist. Luckily there was something in me which wasn't prepared to totally give up, so I 'put it off'. Three weeks later I was in detox, my legs still bandaged. Staying sober has been a fight for life— and I think I'm a lot less likely to act on my feelings if I'm sober. When I feel strongly suicidal, I go into hospital. I have to keep reaching out and talking about it, it feels like an enormous effort to avoid ending it all.

I don't make it up, it's no fun. There are lots of things that seem to make me feel suicidal. Things like the extreme self-blame in my mind, the acute shame, the extreme critic. I guess depressive illness doesn't help. Oh, and the belief I've had that I'm so harmful to others I should kill myself to save them.

All I can say is acceptance of how I feel goes a long way. One night, shortly after memories had come up, I was just so shocked and so down, I grabbed a nurse and told her that I felt I just wanted to die, the pain was too much. And I burst into tears—the despair was almost total. Luckily for me, the nurse didn't challenge me or try to cheer me up. She simply let me express the depth of my pain, as it was, and silently cared. I knew she cared. Getting me to express my feelings allowed the storm to break, and allowed me to go on another day. The despair lessened, the storm passed.

Wendy Nelson

◆

I remember first wanting to die as a little girl of five. My concept of Jesus and his angels seemed a better prospect than the pain of living.

I made my first suicide attempt at the age of 12. Today I am so glad it didn't work. When I first began addressing my sexual abuse, I wished the abusers had killed me. It was such a struggle, but initially I hung in there for my husband and children. Then, wonderfully, I found that I was also worth living for too.

There really is a huge difference between wanting to die and wanting the pain to end. I think it is important to make this distinction. There's also an important difference between healthy sadness and depression. If you think you are depressed, get help. For me to die, I believe, would have been my abuser's ultimate triumph. Always tell someone, even if you think you can't, when you are feeling suicidal.

You are worthy of a life, no matter who did what to you. You can live with abuse, and one day you will find out how brave and wonderful you are for resisting the lure of suicide. Remember that feeling worthless and unable to go on are symptoms of what you've experienced and endured, not statements of truth about who you are.

Louise Plummer

◆

OUR SEXUALITY

Sex is a difficult subject for many survivors of abuse, as it can bring up such potent feelings of fear, disgust, shame, guilt, sadness and anger. Anyone whose physical boundaries have been invaded—whether through physical or sexual abuse—is likely to experience discomfort when thinking about touch. It is hard to enjoy your body when at some time in your life it has experienced not pleasure but the gross misuse of power, and rather than holding memories of nurturing and love it knows pain, shame and sorrow. One of the distressingly powerful aspects of sexual abuse is that our own bodies can come to represent an experience we very much want to forget, but that is meant to be a positive part of many adult relationships. Most of us experienced sexual arousal when abused, and this makes us feel that 'we asked for it', which in turn makes it hard to experience sexual pleasure with our partners as adults without being reminded of our abuse.

It is vital when thinking about sexuality that we do not label ourselves or let others label us or see us as 'the problem', as 'promiscuous' or 'damaged goods'. Those of us who have survived abuse are not 'damaged', we are 'exceptional'. We have an amazing capacity to use our bodies for strength, endurance and survival. Our bodies have helped us to survive, and now it is time for them to be nurtured and honoured in the way they always should have been. That may include not having sex if it does not feel safe to do so, or exploring new ways of relating sexually that do not trigger memories of abusive sexual activities.

This chapter will have special meaning for survivors of sexual abuse, though those of us who have suffered from emotional and physical abuse of any kind will probably also have difficulties loving and caring for our bodies.

I hated my husband kissing me. It always felt as though I was suffocating, and I needed to stop and take a deep breath before continuing our lovemaking. I lived in subconscious fear that he would leave me.

Jan Watson

◆

Sex always felt somehow safer to me if there was an element of weirdness or danger involved. It was as though I was a blind person and my sexuality was my cane—it went slightly ahead of me, sussing things out and protecting me from stumbling and landing face down in the painful reality of feeling my early sexual abuse.

Over the years this pattern has slowly changed. Many things contributed to that. Having a loving partner and good friends who were able to see me clearly was one, working much more physically with my body was another. I think the main thing in the end was that I simply got sick of thinking of myself as a victim. The man who had raped me as a little girl still had power over me as long as I continued to live my life from that place. I decided not to give him that power any more. I realised that I could use my courage to learn to open without fear to my own creativity, compassion and ability to love with or without sex, depending on what I choose.

Linda Savage

◆

It has been very confusing for me as a man working through my abuse in relation to my sexuality. I had to try and move away from a sexuality based on penetration and domination, and I have often felt hurt by a feminist ideology which believes that for men this is all that sex is about. It's not true of all of us!

Richard Kingsley

◆

My abuse happened somewhere up to the age of six. Now I feel divided about sex. On the one hand, it is threatening and just too adult to cope with, and I don't want to know. On the other, I am a prostitute. I was a virgin (apart from the abuse) until I was about 21. By then I was terribly sexually frustrated, but was terrified of involvement. My first partner was someone I met cherry picking. I planned to have sex once and then run away. As it turned out, we stayed together for six drunken weeks. I am 37 now, but that remains my longest involvement.

As for masturbation—I felt so guilty that I didn't start until I was 21, and I used to fear getting caught. I maintained a view of myself as somehow asexual. Romantic hopes and dreams kept me going—long-term infatuations with men who wouldn't or couldn't reciprocate. I would probably have run a mile if they had expressed an interest in me.

Commitment, to me, means being controlled—having my very soul in their hands and being at the mercy of their bodies forever.

I've been in and out of prostitution for about four years now, sometimes loving it, sometimes desperate to avoid it. Going crazy. I've been ashamed of my oscillating, and haven't found anyone to relate to, with this full-on obsession, driven at times by poverty.

I can't comprehend loving sex. To me love and sex don't mix at all. If you love someone, you wouldn't do that to them. I'm very happy to watch the men walk out of my life again after their short visit. No commitment.

I've learnt that love is not the exclusive domain of romance, and I feel in a flow of love with friends, work at ASCA, therapy and AA.

Sex can wait!

Wendy Nelson

✦

The sexual abuse filtered into every area of my life, even though I blocked out my memory of it.

I found that I could leave my body and space out a lot, and I cut myself off from all my feelings. I was totally unaware of my body—whether I was hungry, tired or needed sex. I have had only three serious relationships. The third of these was with the man who is now my husband, who has taught me about love and gentleness. I was totally living in my head and split off from the rest of my body, especially from the waist down, and I felt a strong need to control my husband, my life and all events.

I wouldn't wear make-up or dress really nicely as I didn't want to draw men's attention to me. I avoided sex as often as possible. I felt ugly and didn't like my body, and I started putting on weight when I began working through the abuse; I became afraid of looking attractive or sexy. I always believed men only wanted one thing, and I would try to be friends but not get close in case they wanted sex from me.

I used to resent the fact that I was a girl, and wished I had been born a boy. I felt dirty, smelly and that my body was no good. I have been afraid to have children and be a mother. I felt my sex drive was low and I had difficulty with orgasm although I had experienced it on occasions. One of my greatest fears was of penetration, and I hated it afterwards when my husband ejaculated. I unconsciously had anxiety about sex, and learning to relax was difficult, but I never dared admit this to myself.

It seemed to take forever before I became aroused and I was happy to get it over with. My mind would wander everywhere during sex, and at times I experienced painful body memories. At the time I didn't question it. It is only now, looking back, that it all makes sense to me, and I can see how much it affected me even though my memories of the sexual abuse were repressed. My husband would only have to touch my hair or try to hug me or by accident be slightly rough for me to get really mad and tell him off. I was acting out from my childhood abuse—the signs were always there.

Fortunately when I was remembering my abuse my husband was very encouraging and caring, and said he would not come near me sexually unless I was ready, and this helped me tremendously. I know that in a large part of my marriage I avoided sex for as long as possible. Getting in touch with my sexuality has been rewarding, though I still have to remind myself that it is my husband I am making love to. I am glad to say that I experience orgasm often now. It has been special to have a very sensitive lover who takes care of my needs and fears.

The sacredness of sex is a beautiful way of sharing and expressing our love for one another. I have learned how starved of holding and touching I was. One of my trigger points used to be kissing, but I am now learning to relax and enjoy it. I had endured such violence as a child that I used not to be able even to hold hands without pulling away, afraid of being hurt. I now associate touch with pleasure, and make a conscious effort to enjoy it. I find gentle touch and massage allows me to experience the pleasure of my body. I now understand the issues around touch, but I had no idea about them until I worked on my sexual abuse.

The power of love has helped me overcome the feelings of vulnerability, and allowed me to feel safe to be myself. I am coming to accept my body, even though I am still overweight. My husband's acceptance of me the way I am has helped me to accept the parts of myself that I felt were flawed. I now look back at photographs of myself when I was young and realise that I was attractive, but I never saw it then as I had such a low opinion of myself.

My sexuality is part of spirituality. Sexual abuse is one of the deepest spiritual wounds; we are all sexual beings. It is how we got here, and the sacredness of sex needs to be honoured.

Linda Honey

◆

When my mother found out that I had been abused by my teenage girl babysitter, she scrubbed my penis painfully, making clear her disgust at me. I was informed over and over that female genitals (she used far less scientific terms) were disgusting, and that I was not to touch or play with them.

My teenage arrival into sexual activity amplified this episode. I was very reluctant to touch women vaginally, and for many years

I and my partner were robbed of much natural enjoyment and expression.

After therapy and releasing my anger towards both the abuser and my mother, I gradually moved into a new appreciation of women. Women who resemble my abuser still arouse my interest, though I'm now aware of why!

Taylor Shane

◆

For a long time I felt that my sexuality had been stolen from me. It had been taken without my consent, had been numbed by fear and by my need to protect myself from what was happening to me. It felt as though it did not belong to me, but was merely an instrument for someone else's pleasure.

As an adult I have always felt quite sexual, but when it came to having sex I really didn't enjoy it. I felt incredibly dissatisfied and frustrated with myself because I couldn't enjoy the sexual experiences I was having. I knew something was missing, because I can remember a woman friend describing an orgasm to me, and being pretty sure that I had never experienced what she described. After that day I began to accept that I would never feel much sexually; in my mind I was too 'damaged'.

I saw my role in bed as being the one who gave someone else pleasure, not the one who received it. So I would lie there, acting as though I had never had so much pleasure in all my life, when really I was thinking, 'Two's a crowd'.

One way I began to create a new image of sex was through renaming it. My partner and I called our sex life 'cloud stories' because I could remember enjoying lying on the grass looking up at the clouds and creating images out of them as they drifted by. This peaceful image helped to remove the harshness I felt towards sex, and also helped me to discover that I could enjoy it—and that was such a liberating feeling. It was also a way of acknowledging that this was now a space that was partly mine to create.

Masturbating used to be uncomfortable for me because for a long time I could associate it only with abuse. My father used to tell me to masturbate and think of him; it was a very powerful way to maintain his control over me even when he wasn't around. And it worked: for eight years after the abuse I never touched myself sexually as it frightened me. I now see masturbation as a way of getting to know my own body—and claiming it as mine. As women we are rarely taught to nurture and love our own bodies. Instead we are taught that our sexuality is something given to us through someone else's (supposedly a man's) touch, not something that is already there and can be explored on our own.

As a child I was taught that if I pleased my father sexually he would like me and would not hurt me. I have found it difficult to move away from an identity based on sex and men, but I have been determined to seek an identity of my own, though holding on to it has not been easy. It is important for me to feel the love of my friends; having people around you who know your story can be a great comfort, as they remind you of your strength.

> Men stood beside me
> In front of me
> Behind me
> Within me
> But never with me.
> I want you to stand with me.

Samantha Lee

✦

OUR PARENTING

For some of us, becoming parents triggers memories of the truth of our own childhood. For women this process may begin during pregnancy or when the baby is born (often contributing to postnatal depression); for men as well as women, the innocence, dependence and sensitivity of a small child may be a painful reminder of our own betrayed innocence. We may be bewildered by how difficult we find it to relate to children of a certain age—the age at which we were abused—or the fact that we find ourselves uncomfortable with children of the same gender as our-selves. Children's bodies may seem overwhelmingly vulnerable, or we may be repulsed by them for reasons we do not understand. A child's direct emotional reactions may tap into the raw emotions of our own that we could never express, and of which we learned to be afraid.

It is very hard to be a 'good enough' parent either if our own family of origin was dysfunctional or if other traumatic childhood events have stifled our feelings and our ability to relate naturally. As parents, we may over- or under-compensate, expect our children to look after us when we feel unable to look after ourselves or them, or become abusive parents in our turn. But it is never too late to realise our shortcomings as parents, to explain our difficulties to our children and tell them how sorry we are.

My children still love me despite whatever I may have inflicted on them. They are great people, and as one of them said, 'Mum, we have to break the chain of dysfunction that has gone on in this family'. I have to learn more about who and what I am, and gain an open and frank acceptance of myself. From my children I am trying so very hard to learn to accept my childhood and my role as a mother.

Anne Taylor

✦

It's hard to bring up an emotionally healthy family when there are few close examples to take your cues from. My parents were migrants, and all my aunts and uncles and cousins are overseas. Mum's 'illness' ensured that we didn't have any extended family we could learn to trust and share our growth with.

Diana Beth

✦

I used to spend most of the night in a cold sweat worrying where the children were. My husband laughed at me, but I couldn't stop the anxiety.

Lucy Harlow

✦

My children are remarkable young adults, incredibly angry about what happened to me and the effect this has had on their lives. The deficits of my own childhood are just beginning to come into focus, and I am only able to guess at the impact this may have had on them. They both know they are loved, because they have heard those words all their lives, but they struggle to feel it in their hearts. Following the birth of my first child I suffered from post-natal depression. Just choosing to live was very difficult for the first six weeks, let alone taking care of a new baby. It often felt as though I was looking on from a distance, and I now wonder about that time.

The eldest has always had great difficulty forming close, trusting relationships, and we recently talked about this apparent deficit, wondering about cause and effect. There were times when it was difficult for the children to know who their mother really was, or how the mother-of-the-moment would react. Inconstancy in a parent has potentially disastrous effects on a young child, particularly in developing their ability to trust others and commit themselves as they grow and mature. This had been my own experience. My formative years were full of broken trust and inconstancy, and my heart aches with knowing that I have inadvertently perpetuated this cycle.

The time of my hospitalisation, when I could no longer cope with fighting my memories, was particularly traumatic for the children. The youngest describes it as 'the year I lost my mother—the beginning of the end of my childhood'. He was only six: it must have seemed to him that I had abandoned him. I am haunted by the image of two little people, aged six and eight, sitting on the school fence wondering who would come to take care of them until Daddy returned from the city later in the afternoon. Would anybody come? Who would mother them now, for their mother had clearly deserted them.

Both children have found growing up difficult, and as young adults are now having to take steps to reclaim their own lives. But they are so resilient and forgiving in the face of tremendous odds, so determined to make a success of their lives. I am thankful for their love and support. I grieve for them in their pain, and admire their courage and strength.

Barbara Storey

◆

I was such a fear-ridden child. Everything was a source of danger and a threat: traffic, spiders, strange men, heights, closed spaces, open spaces—the whole world. As an adult I came to realise how unjustified this had been. I was also well aware of how much I had lost because of this approach to life. With no understanding of where my excessive fears had come from, I thought it must have been because I had been given an excess of warnings.

When I became a mother I decided against warnings. I would stand under the double bunk, watching them skylarking on the edge five feet up and thinking, 'Well, what's the worst that can happen? If one of them falls, they could break an arm.' In my mind, breaking an arm was far less harmful than not being able to play. Well, this was a fine attitude, but I didn't notice that I had no sense of proportion about it.

Determined not to inhibit them with needless warnings about the world's dangers, I neglected to warn them at all. They did break their arms, suffer awful accidents, and get themselves into situations that no child should have to extricate themselves from. I was so determined not to do what had been done to me that I did it all again. I left them to face situations that no child should have to face alone—which was, of course, the true source of all my own fears.

Phillipa Brennan

My children have had to grow up a bit more quickly than they should, as they have also felt the effects of the abuse I suffered. They had a mother who did nothing but cry for six months; a mother who couldn't hold it together any more; a mother who was in deep despair and depression. This wasn't the same mother who had raised them. They also felt the absence of aunts, uncles and grandparents from family life. They, as well as I, were pushed out of the family when I disclosed the abuse I had suffered as a child.

Carmol Morley

I think my children must have felt quite rejected. It isn't that I didn't love them, but I couldn't ever show it. When they needed a cuddle, I pushed them away. When they hurt themselves, I found their crying unbearable, and yelled at them to shut up. If they were sad, I felt so awful I couldn't comfort them. I hated to be touched by anybody, as to me touching meant being hit or beaten, and later being abused sexually too. For me, all touch was painful— even the loving touch of my young daughters. It makes me so sad to think of all the hugs we never had. But I've started to change since I realised that I didn't want to pass on my own fears to them; first forcing myself, for their sakes, to touch them on the shoulder, to pat them on the head. Even that was amazing. And slowly it's getting easier . . .

Lily Pike

I was so determined to treat my children differently from the way

I was treated: with fear and punishment and criticism. But it's not so easy in practice. It's hard to know how my children would have differed if I had not been struggling to cope with so many difficulties when they were small. I know it must have affected them, though. When I was feeling really depressed I must have seemed cold, inaccessible, unfeeling towards them: I couldn't respond to their needs when all I could feel was my own desperation and loneliness. As I think of my mother's coldness towards me, so I remember the feeling of yearning and helplessness I experienced when she would not respond.

When he was small my older son was often angry; I'd always felt terribly threatened by anger, and could not let even a small child express any anger at all. To my great regret, I taught him that it was bad to feel angry. He still has the healthy anger and frustration a child feels locked away inside him somewhere—except for what he let loose on his younger brother, who became fearful and depressed. I felt guilty when I finally let my own anger at the bullying (so painful a reminder of what my older brother and sister had inflicted on me) get the better of me. My younger son learned to be the family peacemaker, fitting in with what other people wanted, keeping out of trouble, trying so hard always to be good.

And I pushed them both so hard: I'd never done well enough to please my father and win his approval (and it was only recently that I realised I'd never have gained it even if I'd been the cleverest person in the world, because he was incapable of giving it), but through my children, I went on trying.

What's wonderful is that as I have become healthier, so have the children. As my depressions eased, and my spontaneity and sense of fun returned, so the boys were also able to relax. We're so much happier now than we used to be, and I know that by helping myself I have helped them too.

Candida Hunt

◆

CHAPTER THREE

◆

The effect of our abuse on others

O that 'twere possible
After long grief and pain
To find the arms of my true love
Round me once again!

Alfred, Lord Tennyson, *Maud*

The damage of child abuse is far reaching. It affects not only the survivor but also those we love—our parents and other relatives (if they are not the offenders), our partners and our children.

While we are working on our pain we can become self-obsessed, and often almost impossible to live with. Our nearest and dearest become the hidden victims. If we can help them understand our pain, if we can harness their compassion and support, they may become irreplaceable aids to our recovery.

There are many advice books for survivors, but hardly any for our partners and families. Yet the journey is as unknown, and almost as rough and precarious, for them as it is for us. Neither they nor we know where or when it is all going to end. But while we at least are in the driver's seat (though it often does not feel as though we are), they are often helpless observers. Furthermore, we test those we love, partly because we have so little to give when we are struggling with our pain, and partly to see whether they will stand by us or reject us. With our partners we refuse sex for weeks on end, calling them insensitive even for suggesting it. We stay in bed for days crying. Earning our living, doing the housework, taking the children to school and other normal family activities become impossible.

For a mother, father or loving grandparent the pain is different from our pain, but can be just as bad. They have to suffer the enormous extra burden of guilt, asking again and again, 'Why didn't I realise what was happening? Why didn't I stop it? How could I not have noticed?'

We want partners and parents to read this whole book to help them understand what they are going through with us. Their experience is being repeated all over Australia; they too are not alone. As our supporters, the more they can understand, the more they will be able to help us. Like us, they too need courage and endurance. This chapter has been included to recognise and salute all those who manage to go the journey with us, and particularly those who are still there when we reach the end.

OUR PARENTS

When a child is born its greatest need is for love, care and a safe environment in which to grow up. Most parents are acutely aware of their responsibilty towards their little children, and want to nurture and protect them. Parents feel devastated when they discover that the child's absolute trust in their ability to do this has been betrayed— often by their own partner or by someone else within the family. The pain, the guilt, the sense of failure is enormous; they must carry the burden of these feelings at the same time as supporting the survivor through his or her healing. To make it even harder, parents may think they should ignore their own need for help, sympathy or counselling— perhaps because they believe they deserve to suffer, perhaps because they think it would be selfish to focus on their own distress rather than their child's. Neither is true, and they will be able to help us more by caring for themselves and accepting the fact that child abuse affects everyone.

For survivors the wonderful thing about these contributions is that they are written by parents—and in one case a grandparent—who care so deeply, who truly love their children and are helping them heal. We are grateful for their example; we all wish we had parents like you.

When my child was born, I felt I wanted to love and protect her for ever. I never for one moment dreamed that anyone could ever harm this angel in my arms. This tiny piece of heaven was so innocent, so vulnerable and so dependent. What happened? How could anyone harm something so precious? How can an adult possibly have got pleasure from a child who hasn't even travelled the journey into puberty? It is my child's innocence and trust that have been destroyed. How do you soften their pain and grief? I wanted to be able to do this, so badly. Many times I felt so inept. HOW? How could someone do this?

We must stand by our wounded. We must give them courage, love and hope. How do we know who to trust? How do we pass that on to our children? The burden of their pain as well as our own is so heavy. How much exposure do we need before this taboo subject is dealt with by our politicians, medical people, counsellors, the church, and society in general? This is REAL, this happens. Sexual abuse happens. It cannot be ignored; it will not go away; and it is devastating not only for the victim but also for their family.

Evelyn Miers

◆

On 19 March 1972 a beautiful little girl was baptised in our church. Her two godfathers—her grandfather (my father-in-law) and her uncle (my brother)—took a vow to protect her. But her grandfather soon started to touch her secretly and sexually, and the torment in our home began.

I felt something was wrong, though I couldn't explain my anger or why I felt as I did. Our daughter started to have nightmares, a minor fit and other health problems with no physical cause. I had horrible flashes in my mind of sexual pictures, and as they got progressively worse, so did our daughter's behaviour. No one else could see what I thought I saw. Trying to keep her away from her grandfather was a constant battle, and as I didn't feel able to air my fears with my husband, he could not understand my anger towards his father, why I questioned the fact that his father wanted only to be with our daughter and not with our son, why he took her out in the dark or shut the door to her bedroom, why—red and swollen—she had trouble going to the toilet after his visits. I had difficulty myself facing up to what I believed was happening, and feared that as I was having nightmares too there must be something wrong with me.

The years went by, the same battle going on in our home— yelling at our daughter instead of at her abuser. Eventually I found out that as a little girl I had been abused by my uncles. Perhaps this was what was wrong, perhaps I was imagining what I thought was happening to my daughter because of what had happened to me. I was going out of my mind with worry and with the pain in my own body.

Then I began to wonder why my brother suddenly started to visit us more. But how could I think he was the same? He was a Christian, a leader in his church. As her other godfather, he should have taught her the truth of God, but instead he polluted it with his sexual abuse—abuse of a niece who went to him in trust and told him that her grandfather was abusing her.

My health deteriorated because of my anger, frustration and fear. I could not understand why our daughter spent so much time with our neighbours rather than at home. Then she told me that all the other mothers were good mothers, and were so understanding. I was fighting to keep her safe, to keep her love. Only years later did I find out that the two abusers had always told her that they were the ones who loved her, that her mother had never wanted her and was a very bad mother who had never really loved or cared for her, that her father didn't love her the way they did or he would be doing the same things to her as them, that we loved only her brother and not her. They abused her body and they abused her mind.

When my daughter was 13 years old she finally stood up to them, and also told me what I had so long suspected. She was worried that she might become pregnant by the perpetrators. For the first time I had the truth. But then I did the worst thing I could possibly have done. Because I was a Christian, I told her we had to forgive them, because that is what God would want us to do. How cruel, how stupid, how blind I was to the real truth of God. I added to my daughter's torment instead of helping her. After all those years of horror, I could not handle the truth the right way.

My daughter's struggle was heartrending to watch, while the two abusers went their way as though they had never committed any crime. My husband continued to see his father, still not knowing the real reason why his daughter would not visit her grandfather at his retirement home. He thought there was something wrong with her.

My daughter worked successfully for her degree; the studying took her mind off the pain. She met a young man at the church and eventually married him. She looked so beautiful on her wedding day, but her marriage opened up all the horror of her abuse. Her life became traumatic. Everything fell apart, and her husband was bewildered by what was happening. I was not there to help her through the nights. She tried to kill herself, mutilated herself, smashed things. Thankfully, we had been told about the Salvation Army Family Counselling Service. Praise God for them, for they have given our daughter good, sound, caring counselling. She will continue to need help, but she's a fighter and a survivor.

My husband and I have also had counselling together, which has helped us to handle the effects of the abuse. The anger, the frustration, the hurt, the horror, the disgust and above all, for me, the guilt—all this has to be dealt with. For our beloved daughter there will only ever be love and the desire to see her happy and free from pain. For the abusers, the disgust we feel could only be expressed in words you could not print.

Pat Wagstaff

◆

You have just read my wife's story. As I write, it is two and a half years since I was told that my daughter had been molested, sexually abused from when she was about two until she was 13 years old. This means the abuse ended ten years before I was told about it. I was told then because my daughter was experiencing a lot of stress and problems in her marriage that were directly caused by her childhood trauma.

To say I was devastated would be an understatement. I cannot say I was angry. It was more a great draining of emotion. I felt completely empty. At first it was hard to believe that two people I should have been able to trust, my own father and my brother-in-law, had so dreadfully betrayed our trust in them. We had chosen both of them to be godfathers to our daughter, and my brother-in-law had been best man at our wedding. What bastards.

At the time I was told about the abuse I had been trying to improve my relationship with my father now that he was beginning to show signs of old age. When I tried to confront him with what I had been told, all he would say was, 'We only played the games that she wanted to play'. He didn't want to accept that he was the adult, that my daughter was only two years old when he started, that he had virtually trained her into doing what he wanted from her.

How could I have been so blind as not to see what had been going on? My wife said she had been trying to get me to realise what was happening, without telling me directly what her suspicions were, by getting me to take our daughter to the doctor when she was getting sore. But the doctor always gave some other reason for the state our daughter was in, and it seemed quite plausible to me. Why should I think my own father would do these things to my daughter? It was never in the open—these things never are—

but everyone asks why we let it happen. For goodness sake, we should have been able to trust her grandfather.

I have tried to support my daughter in every way possible, though she cannot understand how I could not have known what was going on. Evidently there were times when I nearly caught them in some compromising situations, but I never did. It seemed to me at the time that they were having a good time together, quite innocently. What a damn fool I was.

As I expect you can tell, I have a lot of self-recrimination, a feeling that I have let my daughter down because of what has happened to her. There is a feeling of loss of family, of a decent family. My feelings towards my father are of disgust and disappointment more than anger. Only when I really think long and hard does anger fill my mind, but I try not to let it get so far that it eats at me. My main concern is what can be done for my daughter to alleviate the trauma she constantly goes through. Yet I know I cannot really help, she must be in charge of her rehabilitation.

She has excelled in her vocation, has obtained a degree and really done well at work. In fact there is a possibility that she is driving herself to forget her childhood, and to mask the effects of what has happened to her. She made the choice to face the police with charges against the perpetrators, and we have gone through the mill of police indifference and having to go to the ombudsman, making contact with the attorney general through our local state member of parliament in an attempt to get some justice for her. My brother-in-law did admit to two of the charges against him, and was sentenced to four months in jail. My father 'ran' to Western Australia to my brother, who supported him. This has made it very difficult to get him to face what he has done. He has been charged with just four counts of sexual molestation after eleven long years of abuse. The law makes it very hard to get justice, but we will fight on for our daughter's sake.

Robert Wagstaff

◆

How can I begin to describe the emotional turmoil that engulfed me when I found out that the child I loved so much was abused by my brother? My first thoughts were to get a gun and splatter him against the wall. I felt so guilty for not being able to do something, I was full of anger. My life was in total upheaval.

I was notified by my other brother that he had found my daughter in a nightclub, scantily dressed and drunk. She had to get drunk in order to be able to tell somebody. The burden had become too heavy.

I can't even begin to imagine the horror she must have felt. She was always a sweet peacemaker, had so many friends, excelled at sport and dancing. The change in her following her abuse was dramatic. She became cold, angry, defensive and detached. She started mixing with people who took drugs, and who were totally unlike her previous friends. She left home, and I didn't hear from her for months. I didn't know how to approach her. Our communication was zero, and although I could see that she was on the path of self-destruction I didn't know what to do about it. I had no support.

When I found out about the abuse I tried to get my daughter to counselling, but she wouldn't go. Then I made an appointment with a counsellor at a major hospital, but I found the counsellor there extremely inept. I had rung various sexual abuse agencies, but they all had long waiting lists, and I didn't feel that the people I had spoken to would be able to give the help that she needed.

My daughter was 16 when she was abused. It took her a long time to realise that it was not her fault. I am so very proud of her. She's now at uni, doing what she loves. She got a late start, but I have total faith that she will make it. I feel like I am her mother again, and she knows that I love her unconditionally and that I'll be there for her no matter what. And she knows that not for a second do I doubt her.

My older son has had great difficulty coming to terms with what happened to his sister. He has lost a much-loved uncle, feels very sad about his sister's loss of innocence; he understands her feelings of betrayal. He is very protective of her and his younger sister. I am trying to come to terms with my heart being torn apart as I watch my daughter and my son in their suffering, though I am glad that they have this beautiful bond of love between them. You can protect and love your children so much, and yet be unable to prevent even the brother you once loved from hurting them in such a devastating way.

Evelyn Miers

◆

On the day I found out that my child had been sexually abused I experienced emotions I had never known before. They ranged from a strange calm at the initial disclosure, through the anger of a parent betrayed, to a feeling that I was adrift in a boat without oars.

When the denial by my nephew came within hours of my accusation, I knew that it was going to be hard to prove what my four-year-old daughter had told me. Everyone seemed more concerned that the exclusive school my nephew attended would find out if the police became involved. No one seemed to care about my daughter. The denial, the lack of compassion for my little girl, left me feeling disgusted with my family, especially my sister's behaviour and her bully boyfriend's threats. I was under a great deal of pressure not to take the matter further, in the 'interests of the family'.

After being laughed at by my sister I did contact the police, which led to accusations from my sister and my father that I was hot-headed, belligerent, a trouble-maker, even deranged. My nephew's denial of something so serious showed me another side of him, the one who had previously been my child's favourite cousin. To me his denial was the most disgusting display of cowardice and weakness. Armed with two lawyers and a QC's opinion my nephew gave a 'no comment' interview to the police. Without some physical evidence or his admitting the offence, the police were not prepared to charge him; likewise, community services did not investigate any further.

Six weeks later my daughter made another disclosure, this time of more deviant behaviour that really sickened me. I realised that my nephew had probably had contact with an abuser himself in order to do what he did to her. Again, the police were contacted but did nothing, and community services told me they could do nothing either unless the boy himself said something about being abused.

Six months after the offence my daughter became ill, with a viral infection that did not clear up. In desperation I eventually took her to a children's hospital, where I sat in a waiting room on two occasions while she was scanned to check for a brain tumour and then a neck tumour. I felt so totally helpless.

When no tumours could be found, she was given massive doses of amphetamines and anti-inflammatory drugs. After two weeks of treatment, her physical deformity moved from one side of her body to the other. The doctors then realised that the cause was psychological. There was a sudden change in attitude in the medical staff when her illness was diagnosed as a physical manifestation of a psychological problem—the trauma of the sexual assault. I was made to feel as if I had wasted their time. The physical pain my child was experiencing was still there, but their compassion was not.

Somehow, I managed to take my child to physiotherapy and psychotherapy two or three times a week over a four-month period, at the same time continuing to study for my degree.

Nine months after the assault, I came face to face with my nephew and my sister's (now ex-) boyfriend. They laughed and jeered at me; my nephew motioned to spit at me, while the other screamed out 'Bitch!' We were in a busy shopping centre, in full view of passers by. I froze, my heart thumping. I thought the six-foot-plus bully boyfriend was going to hit me, so I hurried inside the supermarket—though I forgot everything I needed to buy.

I never thought my nephew would be capable of such disgusting behaviour. He showed no remorse, no guilt, no shame. He was so cocky, so full of himself, flaunting his arrogance that he had been able to get away with what he had done to my daughter. We'll see who has the last laugh.

Anita Webb

◆

My beloved granddaughter Ann looked lovely on her wedding day, so happy, so confident about her future. But the good times did not last. When her daughters were 2 years old and 4 months old she discovered that her husband John was having sex with a 14-year-old schoolgirl. She left him and went to a refuge. He stalked, harassed, threatened and verbally abused her until her life became intolerable. I brought her to live near me at a secret address, but he saw my car one day and followed me to her house. She took an Apprehended Violence Order (AVO) out against him, but the police seemed powerless to stop the abusive phone calls and unwelcome visits.

We moved her again, this time to a country town where my sister and her family live. We changed her name and again kept her address secret. Ann took John to court to prevent him having access to the children, but he appealed and won. She was fearful of his having anything to do with her little girls. There were numerous court cases; her Legal Aid solicitor did a wonderful job looking after her interests, but John had two legal advisers, one of them a QC.

At about this time Ann was notified that John was being charged on five counts of molesting a girl under the age of ten. Like all paedophiles, he was aware that children under the age of eight cannot testify in court—this is why they are so seldom found guilty: they choose very young children. However, he was found guilty, and sentenced to 15 months imprisonment. This was a cause for celebration for Ann and her loved ones, and gave her a break from the strain she had been under for so long.

The children were acting strangely, and my sister drew Ann's attention to this. She sought medical advice, and found that the children had been molested, probably from early babyhood, by their father. This was devastating news to all of us. Apparently he had been abusing them—even the baby—on each access visit. The Department of Community Services (NSW) people counselled and interviewed the older girl, Pam, twice a week. She was very protective of her father, and refused to have a word said against him. I found it very pathetic. She would ask me, 'My Daddy is a good boy, isn't he?' We discovered that he had rewarded her with a can of coke if she was very good—'good' meaning that she didn't tell Mummy or anyone else what he was doing to her. He told her it was 'their secret' and that he loved her 'most in all the world'.

An official from the prison where John is incarcerated demanded that he should have access to the children by phone. After a year and a half of purgatory this was the last straw for Ann. She told me she would kill herself and take her children with her, rather than let him have any contact with them.

Pam was now close to school age, and we were worried that she would be teased about her father. We noticed, too, that mothers drew their children away from her when she tried to do odd things to them, like lifting their skirts, and who can blame them! We tried to change her name but this is not allowed without the father's consent. Ann, a clever girl, decided to have them all, including herself, re-christened with a new name. The school the authorities recommended for Pam was a small one. Some of the pupils were maladjusted, others were physically handicapped or had some other problem. Some of them were bright children. They all needed special care in one way or another. Pam's wounds were invisible, but none the less real.

The principal at the school was wonderful, as was Pam's teacher, and she blossomed. Things began to improve for this little family.

John was in jail, Pam was happy at school, Linda was behaving better. Ann relaxed a little, got herself some things for the house, and began to go out. Then, despite all the caution and the secrecy, John found out Ann's address. Her house was vandalised, her car trashed. She went to a refuge again; threatening messages were left there. From prison, John was getting someone to do his dirty work for him. The family were no longer safe, and had to leave the district.

They left at the dead of night. Their furniture, household things, toys, bikes all had to be left behind. With what she could fit in her little car, Ann drove away to another refuge in another country town. Pam was clutching her school Merit Card in her hand as she got into the car, bewildered, crying that she wanted to stay. She was in despair. She faces a new school now—an ordinary one, this time without any cousins to soften the first day, no special principal, no familiar faces. Exhausted, Ann rang to reassure me. 'We're okay, Nan, don't worry. We'll be settled soon.'

Our family has been devastated by this man. He is without shame, shows no remorse, refuses to admit to having done any wrong. I have written to the attorney general, my MPs and different government departments, pleading for the laws on paedophiles having access to their children to be changed. Surely these people have lost any rights to their children, and should not be given any opportunity to do them any further harm. But John will soon be out of jail, and the family's peace once more in jeopardy.

Ann, from being a strong, healthy, confident young mother, is now a wreck. She has lost her confidence. She is so thin that her clothes hang on her, and her pretty face is lined and anxious. My own health and my husband's is also suffering from the strain and anguish. I feel constantly apprehensive—I'm always expecting a phone call, a letter or a visit from the monster or his friends.

I feel responsible for Ann, and I do all I can to help her and her girls. I will always be here for her, and will do my best to protect her and shield her for the rest of my life. She's a very special girl.

June

◆

My dearest daughter,

How often you are in my thoughts. Your beautiful tender smile, your beautiful eyes that light up with your smile and say 'I love you', without a word needing to be spoken. The special love I feel for you, my first-born child, stays within me forever.

You know how much I miss you. How bewildered and devastated we all are that you were not supported enough to be restored in health so that you could live again. And you were so courageous in your illness. But the medical profession and society were not sensitive to your distress, and disbelieving of the source of your pain.

Since you have died—and I feel this is still something of an unreality for me—there have been so many emotions within me. The despair, guilt, anger fluctuate as I try to come to terms with the fact that you are no longer here. I am guilty because I did not protect you from the unspeakable abuse of your father. Unspeakable because I would never have thought it possible that a father could violate a tiny precious child, and that I could have loved such a person and been blind to such happenings. And yet, there is the truth of it my dearest—I did not know! In my absolute belief in you I have to acknowledge my absolute failure in not protecting you. Please forgive me.

And while you were ill and as gradual realisation of the nature of your illness unfolded, it became a nightmare I shared with you, but you carried the pain of it alone for so long. And so there are the inevitable 'if onlys' going round and round in my mind. If only I had known sooner, maybe I could have done more to restore your will to live. If only your partner had told me of the depression you were suffering following the death of Nan and Pop, maybe I could have been more supportive. But the two of you seemed to be so 'together' it would have felt presumptuous to intrude. I now ask myself how I could have been around you more.

You know, my darling, I look at photographs of you and you are smiling, or pensive, or clowning, and my heart aches and love for you wells up in me. You are so wonderful, so beautiful in my eyes, and you always will be.

But I miss you so, we all miss you so. How I would love to hold you, hug you, give you strength. We could have made it together, my darling. Could have . . . If only . . .
Love from
Mum

Margaret

◆

I can only tell you that I will never forgive myself for not protecting my child. I know people mean well when they say, 'It was not your fault'. But if I could not protect her, who could?

Diane McNamara

◆

I am not only the mother but also the daughter, sister and wife of victims of child abuse. Although I was not directly abused myself, the abuse throughout my family has irrevocably damaged my life too. When I was reunited after 36 years with the son I had been forced to give up for adoption as a young unmarried mother, I found a desperate, disintegrating man who looked to me to put him back together again. I had not been able to protect those closest to me earlier in my life; now I was determined to support him, a survivor of emotional, physical and sexual brutality.

Once my son knew that I could handle things, that I was non-judgmental, that we could discuss any subject and I was not going to flee in horror or reject him, then trust developed. The tests and trials he subjected me to were excruciatingly painful and made me exceedingly angry at times. We had our arguments and disagreements, but continued the dialogue. I came to realise that as I was the parent it would always be up to me to give him what he needed, even though he was unaware and oblivious, as any child is, of the pain he might be inflicting on me. I learned that when he said, 'Is it all right for me to love you?' what he really meant was, 'Is it all right for me to trust you?' If he had used the word 'trust' he would have exposed his own vulnerability, and that he could not do.

Lorraine Gee

◆

Being the mother and supporter of an 11-year-old child survivor of organised sadistic (ritual) abuse is an emotionally demanding full-time job. My daughter told me of the abuse after I had separated from her father. The reality is that I am caring for many very damaged invisible children, whose ages range from newborn up to the age she is now. This is really pioneering parenting. During the most difficult year there really needed to be two or three of me to cope with my daughter's emotional needs. She was waking up at about 8 p.m. wanting breakfast, lunch or dinner, and going to sleep at about 8 a.m. I tried to be there for her (awake) as much as possible.

My daughter has an unknown number of parts or personalities, some programmed into her by the perpetrators and some she created herself. The parts created by my daughter helped her through, and out of, the severe abuse.

My caring role limits opportunities for social and supportive networks. I do not have a sense of really belonging anywhere. There are few recovering survivors as young as my daughter, so we are very isolated. This is especially so as my demanding work is invisible and mostly unacknowledged. Sometimes I feel so much sadness and loss I am overwhelmed by grief. However, even with all the damage and destruction to my children and me, my daughter and I have emerged triumphant.

My daughter has asked me to say on her behalf that she is steadily recovering, thanks to her own strategies combined with my love and support. She also has an experienced and compassionate therapist, and we can ring Rape Crisis phone counsellors when she is in crisis. We try to live in the present and focus on our inner strength of spirit and courage. I read *Beyond Survival* and we get a lot of comfort from knowing through the magazine that we are not alone in our struggle.

Debra Lee

◆

I felt incredible guilt for many years. My daughter Liza came to me when she was eight years old and told me that Poppy (her grandfather) had touched her. I confronted him and he denied it, saying, 'How could you ever think this of me?' At the time she had thrush, so I decided that perhaps she had meant he was putting the cream on her. I loved my father very much, we were such a close family. My parents lived with us, the kids loved them. I had never heard of child abuse then.

With hindsight I can't believe how stupid I was. He used to sit with her on the lounge with a blanket over both their laps. His hands were under the blanket, so he was probably abusing her even while we were in the same room. I'm over my guilt now. It took a few years, but I love my daughter and am doing everything I can to help her have a life.

Sally Hilman

◆

Sally knew for two years, and didn't tell me what was going on. One day, when Liza had been really awful to me for no reason, I said, 'What the hell is going on with you? Something's up that you're not telling me!' So they told me. I felt such rage towards my father-in-law I felt like killing him, and I also felt betrayed by Sally. I knew that she hadn't seen him for a couple of years, but he was stealing money from my business and I thought it was because of that. It seemed a good enough reason. Sally explained later that she hadn't told me because I would have done something stupid and how would she and Liza have coped when they were already feeling so fragile? She's right, too—I would have.

My daughter is such a beautiful girl. He's scum. I'm over my feelings now, I just want Liza to get better.

Harry Hilman

◆

I prayed for a husband who did not smoke, or drink to excess, was of the same religion and was not a womaniser. I also prayed that I would have a happy marriage.

I was given what I prayed for—for about 36 years. Then it became like a beautiful piece of furniture that was riddled with white ants. My three daughters recovered their memories and accused their father of heinous crimes towards them. This meant that my marriage had not been happy after all; I had just thought it was.

I had not the vaguest notion that any father—and especially my husband—would abuse his children. Yet there had been signs, if I had only known how to read them. I could never understand why my darling little children were so often unhappy, and continued to be as they grew up—particularly the son who killed himself.

My daughters often seem all right on the surface, but they are afflicted with an obscure pain so bad that it nearly sends them mad. At times this hidden pain overwhelms their beautiful natures, so that all outsiders can see is them expressing pain in its various ugly forms.

I wish I could be in three places at once to help my daughters because I am their number one support. That does not mean that I can help them much, because I have to admit that sometimes I am a bad part of their memories. Imagine back to the time when they were little, their cries for help. 'Mummy! Mummy!', and wondering, 'Why isn't Mummy here to help me?' And he told them lies, said, 'Mummy told me to hurt you,' and threatened them.

Most of the time, I am comforted that my presence is of great value to my daughters. My heavily pregnant second daughter sits on my lap, her head on my shoulder, with my arms around her while she cries for all that she lost with the pain peculiar to recovering memories. My other two daughters periodically ask to be hugged, but generally they bear their pain in solitude (or is that loneliness?).

One daughter is in her forties, two are in their thirties. Recently I grieved for all the lost opportunities, and because I could not go back in time and have them again as little children who I could nurse and hug to kiss their pain away.

I have endured much to face the horror of what happened to my little girls. The truth of their memories is proved when I compare how they used to be (very depressed and unhappy) and how they are now (coming along very nicely). With the release of their memories of horrible, painful events they experience a joy, a love of themselves that they never had before. It does my heart good to see them improving, and leading a more 'normal' life—sustaining relationships for longer, holding down a job instead of constantly being sacked, being far closer to each other, handling disappointments better, communicating positive messages to themselves, not to mention their greater beauty and sweeter voices.

F. Hayden

◆

OUR PARTNERS

Helping a survivor through their healing is an incredible test of a relationship. Our partners are our lifeline, and we test it and them to the limit. The journey is difficult, and on the way we sometimes discover that the relationship is not strong enough or healthy enough to sustain us, and we must continue it alone. But the partners who stick with you, who share and help you through your pain, are worth their weight in gold. Their patience is eventually rewarded with a deeper, stronger, better relationship. It is notable how much faster survivors heal when they have a supportive partner to share their struggle. We have encouraged contributors to this section to write at some length, because it is rare to find accounts of their experiences, and their insights are so valuable.

It was a near-death experience that caused my wife to start recovering memories of abuse in her childhood. Had we never had any inkling before that? Well, in retrospect, I guess there had been some indications in the course of our 23 years together, but really they were little signs only: unreasonable, irrational fears at times, about all sorts of things; being over-protective of our children; contrasting vulnerability and aggressiveness—but that was all. Neither of us thought there was anything hideous lurking in the past. Facing death in a runaway vehicle was the trigger. Over the following months she started reliving traumatic childhood events in the form of flashbacks. Those moments were really scary, but we agreed it was better to open up the old wounds than try to cover them over. And anyway, you really don't have any choice once it's started—you just have to confront your past, despite the emotional rollercoaster it brings. We've been walking on broken glass for two years now, and I think we've still got a way to go, but there's no other way to handle it successfully. It takes guts, and she's been extraordinary.

How have I coped? I have to admit it's been tough. I've been on overload too. But I'm a long-distance runner and cyclist by training, and I guess I have stamina and a high tolerance of pain. In those sports you get to accept that you have to take the pain for any long-term gain.

I've often been unsure of what to say in particular situations, of what to do for the best. I've always tried to be supportive, to make her feel sure that I'll be around no matter what. You have to take one day at a time, you have to wake up every morning with a strongly positive attitude, just so you can make it through the day. It takes real self-discipline.

The advice I would give a partner is: read as much as you can about recovering traumatic memory and all the best books on child abuse. Find a Bessel van der Kolk video. Immersing yourself in the subject will help both of you.

Alan Robinson

✦

I want to say at the outset that I am really proud of Joseph. It's not easy to face a hurtful, horrific past. Sometimes I marvel at his strength and courage and sheer determination to face the past, deal with it and move on. Usually therapy for such trauma takes anywhere from three to ten years. I myself can only live one day at a time. If I thought I had another nine years to cope, I'd go crazy. My faith in God sustains me, and he gives me only enough strength for one day.

I met Joseph's counsellor and had about half an hour with him. It was great to be able to ask questions, to understand a bit more of where Joseph's at, what his counsellor's approach is, what I can do to support him. I came away most encouraged. Joseph is making great progress and seems generally to be getting better in himself as he faces the memories that are surfacing—except when he has his off days. I guess it's going to be up and down for a while yet.

Some days I forget that he's going through therapy for the worst abuse possible—physical, sexual, emotional. The police have even been involved because his father has been responsible for so much abuse, none of which has gone to court. When it all came out I freaked at first. I didn't want to accept it. I had to keep the home running smoothly, while working part-time, helping in our business, and carrying out the many duties and pleasures of motherhood.

On Joseph's down days I feel quite shut out. I used to take this personally, but I'm learning to give him the space he needs. He cannot give anything to me when he's like that, so I just have to get on with it. I feel there's nothing I can do to help. For example, one night around dinnertime he said, 'I feel wiped out, I need to go and lie down'—total emotional overload. We have two young children, and I had an extra one staying that night, so with my husband a write-off and me wondering what he was going to be like when he woke up, I had to organise the kids and also deal with my own emotions—tension, frustration, anger at his father, teariness, loneliness, fear. Joseph got up several hours later. By then I was ready for bed, but he wanted my company. So I have to be there for him when he's out of it, and also there when he wakes up. It's not that I don't want to, but it's hard to cope with sometimes.

I suppose I'm learning just to accept whatever is happening and to understand more what he's feeling and going through. It's so much harder for him than for me, though I find comparisons quite unhelpful. I can acknowledge that it's been hell for him, but not with empathy because I haven't been abused—he doesn't expect me to understand, only survivors understand each other—but I still need validation that it's hard living with a survivor at times. He has said I can go if I like, I don't have to hang around. Rather than feeling released, though, I feel that all the responsibility is back on me. Often I don't feel like a wife. I don't feel cherished and nurtured in the way that only a husband can do—indeed like he used to. I feel like I'm just a friend. I'm hoping intimacy—physical, emotional and spiritual—will be restored in the future. Friends are great, but they're no substitute for a husband.

I've just started seeing a counsellor myself which is helping me tremendously. She understands what Joseph is going through, and it's great spending time with her. The other thing that has been essential was to build up support around me—a few friends I can ring at any time, people who can help with the kids, etc. I often write in a journal too, which helps—just to write all my feelings out: the anger, frustration, fear, sadness, insecurity, weariness, injustice. Sometimes I stress out about whether he'll be able to keep functioning and bring in an income. I help where I can, but I'm limited with a young family. Again I trust God to take care of us.

Recently I decided to 'get a life', so to speak. I can't focus exclusively on what Joseph's going through. I need to reach out and want to have a positive impact on other people's lives. Perhaps I can offer hope or a listening ear to them. Joseph is quite antisocial much of the time. It takes so much energy for him to function and stay in control that there's not much left for socialising. Our physical intimacy has also suffered a great deal. Because he was repeatedly abused sexually, as memories surface, sex repulses him. I want to be patient and stick by him, because the people he trusted in the past violated that trust—and I love him and hate to see him suffering as he is. I guess it's teaching me a whole new side to what unconditional love is all about!

When Joseph did try to give himself physically to me on my birthday, the next day he couldn't bear to touch me, and was really out of it. This was pretty painful for me. He was totally wiped out—the experience brought up a whole lot of painful memories for him. I found this extremely hard, feeling very angry that he couldn't forget about himself for even one day and think about me. But he couldn't. We didn't talk about it for a few days. I took it all personally until we communicated and I realised afresh how hard it is for him. He feels as though there's a war constantly going on inside him, that he wants to burst into tears much of the time.

Don't give up on the survivor you're living with. You don't gain anything from running away. Love them. Really love them—it's not their fault they were abused. They're doing something about the hurt done to them. Be determined to help them overcome the evil done to them with good. Ask how you can best support them, and do it. Accept that it will be hard, really hard at times, for both of you. Get support, even counselling, read relevant books. Now is not the time to be independent, thinking that you can make it on your own. Be someone who doesn't violate their trust as others have. People at the other end tell me it's worth it, and I for one want to believe them. Never stop hoping that things are going to get better.

Jenny Scott

◆

The circumstances of recovering memories are quite bizarre—little of one's life experiences can prepare us for it. My wife's first recall of memories started months after she became ill. The sickness was physical, not emotional: extreme tiredness, inability to eat, specific body pains. Naturally, we relied on our wonderful GP friend to solve it. When this failed, she went into hospital—and Macquarie Street's finest tested her for just about everything. Our biggest fear was that it might show up the Big C. But there was nothing. Then the specialists recommended investigative surgery—and we baulked.

Back we went to our GP, now feeling really concerned. What do you do with a seriously ill patient who has nothing wrong with her? Of course, you take her to Noosa. But nothing changed. She went up in a wheelchair, and came back in one.

In the following weeks, logically, we moved to an alternative healer, who posed the question of whether she'd been abused as a child. How ridiculous. At the age of 47, you'd *know*, wouldn't you? Her family had never said anything, but—well, you do have to consider any possibility.

We realised later, much later, that the essential factor in making progress was finding a totally safe, supportive environment for her to investigate her ghosts. We were lucky in finding that special place, that special therapist. But we were quite unprepared for the trauma, the disruption, the shattering impact of recalling horrific childhood events. The frequent tears, the suicidal feelings, the bewilderment, the denial.

In her case the abuse had been confined to a single week of her life at the age of five, and the perpetrator was not a family or extended family member. In that sense we were very lucky indeed. The involvement of family, or abuse over a sustained period, must have unimaginable, hideous, overwhelming repercussions.

Nevertheless, for rational, mature adults the initial months of recovering memories were quite bizarre. Neither of us knew anything about the subject, we'd never heard of *The Courage to Heal*. I learned more slowly than she did, maybe because I was not the one going through it, and I made all the predictable mistakes, asking, 'If it's so painful going back, is it the sensible course?', 'Can't you just dig it all out in one session, rather than drag it out endlessly?', 'Is it sensible to put your trust totally in the therapist?', 'Are you really making progress? You seem to be getting worse'.

I became involved in the process of her healing, discussing the healing journey with the therapist—and realised I should have been there at the outset. I also realised I couldn't remain a neutral observer in the issue of recovered memory. Against the quietly sceptical friends—isn't it surprising how everyone has an opinion?—I had to be totally supportive and shielding of my wife, which meant reading everything I could on the subject. I even tried to provide substantiation of her memories, as the ultimate response, but found that the passage of 42 years and the death of her mother made it impossible. If only . . .

We're through the tunnel now, and realise how profoundly the experience has changed our lives. Fortunately, in a very positive way.

Rod Phillips

◆

In the beginning I found it difficult to come to terms with my partner's abuse. I wanted to believe that what I was being told simply wasn't so, that none of it was happening. I put it into the too-hard basket. Over time I found to invalidate someone else's reality was the worst thing I could do. The fact that it came up was bad enough for my partner, without me putting my self-righteous judgments on it as well. As my partner became more deeply involved with her abuse and became immobilised, I tried to help her as best I could. Difficult feelings about incidents in my own childhood that I had never dealt with were also coming to the surface, so whenever my partner's feelings came up I would try to get her out of them. That was a bad mistake, but if you've never dealt with your own feelings, you can't help anyone else with theirs.

It's been more than three years now since this all started, and we have both come a long way since then. My partner is actively finding more and more ways to get other people to support her, and has been to see various government ministers and departments for more funding and more services that are vitally needed. I have become more supportive of my partner, though it has taken some time to reach this level. I guess what all survivors want is to be heard. I have found this difficult, but I know that being listened to and believed is the most beneficial aid to recovery anyone can receive. Don't doubt with your mind—feel with your heart.

David Honey

◆

My wife's battle with recovered memories started about five years ago. It followed weeks of poor sleep and nightmares. We knew something was wrong, but we didn't have the faintest idea of just what it was.

Then it really started. Early on we realised it involved her grandfather, and he was still alive at the time. This brought more problems. What do you do, confront the perpetrator? Share your trauma with the rest of the family? For the best of reasons we decided we wouldn't burden other family members—our great concern was that if they handled it badly, my wife would be abused all over again.

She didn't get professional help in the beginning, and that was our first big mistake. She made it a full-time commitment, and devoured books on all the related subjects: self-esteem, trust, depression. It was hard, impossibly hard for her—and all I could do was be supportive.

Like most men I'm a problem-solver with a 'let's fix it' attitude, but situations like ours don't respond to that approach. I found it incredibly frustrating. I didn't know what to do, to be honest.

Events evolved daily, and developed a momentum of their own. Life was pretty disastrous. I was trying to be supportive, working 60 hours a week, and not sleeping. She was heading for a total breakdown. It was only later that she sought professional help. Once that started, though, we made incredible progress.

Mistakes? There's no manual about confronting child abuse, but early professional help is one key move—find a psychologist who's had experience counselling survivors. Another is to follow your own instincts. Patience is another. Of course it's a trial by fire for any marriage. Happily for us, it's been a reinforcement. There's now a great sense of security, because of all that we've shared.

Stephen McMurray

◆

I think the first indication I had that my partner carried some traumatic memories was when she wouldn't take my hand to cross the street. A simple act in itself, one which doesn't necessarily carry any connotations of sexual advances, but was somehow very confronting for her.

When her memories started to peek out from behind the screen she had created to protect herself, I was frankly very happy. I knew there was something in the past, but unless she herself recognised it, we couldn't move ahead. From that moment on, we travelled the healing path together. Sometimes it would be days before she could talk about her therapy session. It was difficult for her because her experience had previously been invalidated—'You're just imagining it', etc. Sometimes it was for fear of losing me. She would worry, 'It might be too much', and 'Will he still want me when he knows about Dad?' and 'Will he be able to keep it secret?'

I can say that our relationship grew stronger. It may sound odd, but our love grew through our sharing very intimate feelings of hate and love for the perpetrator. I learnt that my partner was a multiple, and over a period of some years I found she had seven, quite distinct personalities locked up inside. I learned first to identify each personality, which made it easier to cope. There might be a very aggressive answer, which I thought was unwarranted until I realised it was someone else talking. I learned to 'hear' that personality, and to try to understand his or her point of view. Yes, there were two male personalities in addition to two children, a seductive woman, and a forceful personality called 'achiever'.

For me it was absolutely crucial to share everything along the way. The therapy sessions, when my partner could not drive home because of some new revelation, the times when we couldn't make love or even touch because the memory blocked that touching, the sudden change in personality that left me dealing with another person until I realised a switch had taken place. It sounds confusing, but it was not if I understood each step along the way of healing. I had support from the therapist, who realised that there was a threesome involved—that is, that I was important too. There were times when I could talk directly to the child or one of the other personalities. The voices were different, the energy very different; the understanding of the little one was childlike and very beautiful.

I'm glad I didn't continue my life as if nothing had changed. I'm glad I met and talked at a soul level with my partner, and sometimes allowed my own little five-year-old out to play as well. I can say that this journey with my partner has been the most beautiful thing in my life. Through the journey I have also come to understand myself better. There were times when my needs were not being met and it was important to say so, both for me and for my partner. It was confirmation that we both had needs and that the healing process is a two-way thing.

Murray Johns

As the partner, it is possible to become vicariously traumatised by what the survivor is going through. It is painful to hear traumatic stories about someone you love. You will probably need your own personal therapy group or a strong support network, as much as the survivor. It is a long-term role and can be exhausting and frustrating, but also incredibly rewarding. Changes do not, and cannot, happen overnight. There might be times you want to walk away from it all, and yet something keeps you in there. Partners need to be honoured as much as survivors for struggling with the healing process. For many, over time both lives have changed dramatically for the better. If you are still struggling, I hope you both have much loving support and encouragement in your journey.

Zoe Hagon

What is it like to be the partner of a ritual abuse survivor? How do you react to the knowledge that the person you live with has participated in or even led rituals of terrifying violence? How do you react to the denial of all these events that continues to place your partner in danger from her family? How do you react to the continuing persecution by the abusers—the drive-by tooting, the whistles, the following of your car, the people over the fence or outside the house and workplace, the strange messages or noises on the answering machine? Cult members do not wear uniforms, have no distinguishing characteristics and go to great lengths to be invisible.

I have no easy answers to any of these questions, but I have learned to live with each of them and now know that things do get easier as together we move farther and farther out of the cult's shadow. What a process it has been.

As a survivor of ritual abuse, my wife revealed many personalities during her healing journey. I enjoyed the company of the 'children' inside her, and admired their courage. Their trust and friendship was, and still is, very special to me, and it made me realise just how much I enjoy being a father. We spent many hours together watching gentle, non-violent cartoon stories and eating popcorn, shopping for toys, walking on the beach and talking about life in the 'up-world', the world that is not cult. Time spent with them was precious beyond words, but always tinged with a sadness that came from knowing the terrible experiences that they had lived through and survived.

Their joy and determination to overcome the past helped me to move forward, not to become trapped in the past and allow those events to overwhelm me. I guess that I have learned to live with the uncertainty, and to become something of an expert at navigating through a world of shadows and fog—proof is so hard to find.

I see nothing remarkable in what I have done. I guess that, despite everything, I still have fun, and we still had fun together as a couple even at the most difficult times. Being able to see the lighter side and have fun even in the most frightening situations or darkest moments definitely helped.

Would I change anything? On my dark days I think that maybe the whole thing was too hard and the toll on my health, my peace of mind and my life was too much for any one person. On my better days I can see past the things that annoy me, though being stalked still annoys the hell out of me.

Roy Stevens

◆

Over the last three years or so, the story of my life and of my marriage has been tied up in many ways with dealing with my wife Lydia's memories of the abuse she experienced in childhood. The reality of Lydia as a survivor has been a big part of my life.

Lydia and I had been very close in the years leading up to the recovery of her memories of abuse. We had worked very hard at building our relationship, at sharing things with each other, and at being able to talk with each other. When her memories began to return, we shared them at first. I recall a night when the awareness of some kind of overpowering evil was so strong I had to get her breathing again so she could fight what was attacking her. But as time went on, and as the memories became stronger and clearer, I was no longer kept in touch with what was happening. I say it like that because it wasn't a deliberate attempt to shut me out, but the sharing was just not there any more. And in the end it happened fairly quickly. There was suddenly a huge area of life that was not open between us. This was Lydia's stuff—it was definitely not my stuff. Something was suddenly cut loose between us, and I was somehow adrift. I knew then, as I know now, that there were reasons for that, and indeed that some of the reasons were actually in me and my lack of understanding or my inability to give Lydia what she needed. But I was still adrift.

I knew from the beginning of Lydia's remembering that I wanted to support her. One thing that I didn't know was that supporting her would often seem to mean that I would be carrying on in the dark. I often didn't really know what was happening for her, or how she was responding to things, or indeed whether she was responding to me or to something in her counselling and her memories. I kind of fumbled through, did the best I could, and trusted to some kind of luck that I wasn't driving her away from me, or back into some form of horror that I couldn't even guess at. I did things with the kids, and tried as best I could to keep everything going in the house, and wondered what this evening, or the next morning, might bring. We might be lovers, or I might earn only a grunt of acknowledgment. And often I could not predict what it might be.

One thing I found really valuable was a book called *Allies in Healing* by Laura Davis. She writes of the things that partners experience. It gave me some answers, and some hints to find my own answers, and it helped me to know that I was not alone in what was happening.

I found, as time went on, that I had to choose to be more responsible for myself. This had more to do with attitude than behaviour. I had to learn to say, 'This is who I am and this is what I've done, and I'm content with that.' I had to allow my own affirmation of myself to be enough. I could not expect Lydia to affirm me, or to take on my stuff, or to be my sounding board. She was too caught up in her own work on her abuse issues to do that. If I needed affirmation I had to be able to give it to myself or to find it from someone other than her.

As Lydia and I found we were becoming less in touch in the big and personal things that were happening, I found myself needing more and more to emphasise my trust of her. Even when we first began to go out together, she had pointed out to me that trust is the crux of a relationship, and as her memories came back and her counselling proceeded, and she was working on things and changing and putting new things into her life, I simply had to trust her. She began to go out in the evenings to survivors' meetings, to do courses, to study counselling, and in some ways these things were threatening because they were new and I had just to trust that Lydia still wanted to be married to me. The trust was hard, especially when it became clear that it was not helpful to Lydia when I said, 'I love you'. The idea of love had been part of the way she had been groomed for abuse in her childhood. I simply had to trust, and carry on.

Lydia's therapy meant that we had to make financial sacrifices. At times I was angry and resentful about that; I had to look at the priority of Lydia's therapy and deal with my anger and resentment in ways that kept it private and belonging only to me. It would have added to the abuse Lydia had suffered if I laid my anger or resentment on her. One place where I found that particularly hard was in my own need for therapy and for someone I could talk with about what was happening with me.

One thing that has been important for me—as a way of caring for myself and meeting some of my needs—has been to join a local gym. It was like opening a window to look in another direction away from all the things that had been so overwhelming, tied up with family and abuse and responsibility. It was something just for me, that I did alone, that I was safe and comfortable with. I was able to feel good about myself.

Looking back, since Lydia began remembering, I am aware of many benefits. I know I have become more sensitive. I'm in touch with feelings, both my own and other people's. My respect for the women's movement has grown, as has my respect and admiration for Lydia as I see what she shows me of her struggle. I am immensely proud of her and the work she has done for herself, seeking and finding the growth and change she has needed. I know how fortunate I am to be married to her. If I were to sum it up, I guess I would say that I have become aware of a gentle strength in myself that I like and that I think helps me get on a bit better in the world as well. Today, it's a nice place to be.

James Grey

◆

Did I really say at the outset of Helen's therapy that I 'would listen for three weeks, seven days a week'? If I did, I was incredibly naive. It took Helen nine months of weekly therapy to reach the actual sexual assault, then up to twice a week for five months to begin to deal with it.

At the time Helen was confronting her past, my support was complicated by my parents' death. We both had lives to grieve—

I the end of my parents' lives, and Helen the damage that had been done to her own.

Helen's emergence from her pain found expression in gestures of rediscovered control over her well-being, and eventually well-being became kinship with a lover.

Guy Sherborne

◆

Cathy and I were married at 25. At that time she had clear recollections of sexual and other forms of harassment from her older brother, but no memories of sexual abuse. The trigger to her process of understanding herself was the death of both her parents only a few months apart, and—at about the same time—her pregnancy with our third child. She began working through the way messages about herself originating from her childhood were affecting her life now. Ingrained messages about her worthlessness had to be separated from truth and reality, and she showed enormous tenacity. As she worked at her own issues she developed the ability to listen and to help others work through their own painful memories, and I was amazed at how readily people could open up and unburden themselves to her.

Ten years into this process Cathy first began to recall the sexual abuse. She knew there was something big and painful yet to be uncovered. Gradually the pictures began to become clear and to join together to form coherent memories. It was long and painful for her. After a while she found a skilled counsellor and began to make rapid progress—if you can describe a process stretching over several years as rapid. She has been able to get confirmation from relatives of some of the events she remembers.

There was a time when I felt furiously angry at Cathy's parents. Her father and brother were both her abusers, and her mother had collaborated in various active and passive ways. The abuse had started when Cathy was four years old, possibly even younger. My rage was so fierce that if the parents had not already been dead, I could easily have put myself in jail by killing them.

Accepting and supporting Cathy in her healing process was important, but not terribly difficult, until I realised that I needed to change the way I treated her. It became obvious that I couldn't separate my own behaviour from her abuse memories and her healing process. When I feel threatened, insecure and disapproved of, my reaction tends to be to withdraw into my shell, and I become almost unable to speak. (This is quite a contrast with when I am feeling confident.) While I am feeling insecure, the one comfort I seek is close physical contact. But physical contact in silence was part of the pattern of Cathy's abuse, and my behaviour is often a trigger for some of her defensive mechanisms. I, in turn, can easily interpret some of her reactions as disapproval, driving the spiral down further. We both understand that this kind of circular dance needs to be broken, and that it isn't possible for one of us alone to change the pattern—we both need to learn new steps.

It has been surprisingly difficult to learn new ways of responding, and I still have a long way to go. The damage done to me in my upbringing was modest compared with the severe damage done to survivors of abuse, so if changing my patterns is difficult, how much more difficult it must be for survivors. My admiration for those who work through to a real degree of healing is enormous.

It has taken me quite a few years to acknowledge to myself what should probably have been obvious in the first place:

- A survivor can never recover to become a person who was not abused as a child. It is useless to pin your hopes on that kind of recovery.
- A victim can become a recovering survivor, but the time this can take can be measured in years.
- The healing process never ends, and even after major gains have been achieved, there is always more work to come and more issues yet to surface.
- Recovering survivors have a strong contribution to make to the

lives of others. 'Normal' people tend to treat them as though the giving is always from the 'normal' to the survivor, but there is a great deal of room for the giving to come from survivors to others too.

Phil Barrett

✦

There are times when I think the greatest barrier to my partner's journey of recovery from a childhood characterised by abuse is me. Several years into our marriage, as the light of awareness began to shine upon years of violence and shame, there were times when depression seemed to take over. As the process began there was pain. Pain as she remembered and came to terms with the past. Pain as she confronted the present. Pain as she considered the next dark doorway to be opened to the light.

For me there is also pain. Pain as I am confronted by my partner's past abuse. Pain as my own presuppositions and beliefs are challenged by a new reality. Pain as our relationship has had to change to accommodate and to comfort a background and a person neither of us has ever really met before. Yet beyond this is still another challenge: for me this is not a journey of revealing past experiences and abuse, but a re-education of what life so often is really like—if only we'd look.

It is still a journey for me, and each day I have to decide afresh if I will continue on it. Sometimes that's hard, but if the strength and willingness of my partner to reveal the shadows of her experiences remain as a guide for me and my own subsequent journey, then the path is before me. All I have to do is travel along it.

David Mitchell

✦

CHAPTER FOUR

✦

Less acknowledged forms of abuse

What lies behind us and what lies before us are tiny matters compared to what lies within us.

Anon

It is almost always difficult for we survivors of child abuse to feel that our memories and perceptions of our childhood are true, that our feelings are valid. There are some groups of survivors for whom this is made even more difficult because people find it impossible to believe in their form of abuse.

Society is finding it hard enough to believe that any child abuse is as prevalent as it really is; the credibility gap widens dramatically when it comes to abuse of boys, abuse by women, and the extremes of sadistic and ritual abuse. We have included this chapter because we want to do something to redress the balance. So, although there are throughout the book accounts of memories and of healing by men who were abused as children, and by both men and women who were abused by women, abused sadistically, abused in rituals, here they talk more specifically about their experiences. Their silence has been the greatest; their voices deserve a particular place in which they can now be heard. Readers who may until this point have feared that the book does not apply to them because their own abuse falls into one of these categories will, we hope, find comfort and validation here: this book is also for you.

MEN WHO HAVE BEEN ABUSED

Until the 1980s the subject of physical and sexual abuse of male children was largely ignored. Corporal punishment was regarded as an acceptable method of discipline—'I was beaten as a boy and it never did me any harm, in fact I'm sure I deserved it' being a common response—while the question of sexual abuse was simply not considered. Most of the research since then has been undertaken in the United States, where many scientific surveys and academic studies have been conducted. The results have been published in a number of well-regarded books and journals. The evidence in Australia is more anecdotal at this stage, but it is likely that the same pattern of abuse exists here as has been uncovered in the United States. Recent investigations of the NSW Royal Commission have highlighted the abuse of boys but have also rather skewed public debate on this matter. Rumours about politicians, priests, judges and other public figures forming homosexual rings and preying on young boys make lurid headlines but obscure the ordinary reality which is that the vast majority of boys, as with girls, are abused by members of their own family.

A boy is no more capable than a girl of resisting inappropriate physical or sexual invasions by an adult or an older adolescent. He's rarely phys-ically stronger, he's emotionally no more mature, and the adult-child power differential is no different. Yet it is very hard to convince people that many boys as well as many girls are abused in Australia. Why? Prob-ably because it's an unpleasant truth we don't want to acknowledge. But arguing about the prevalence of abuse of boys in Australia is not really the important issue. What matters is that it should be recognised for the awful crime it is, and that public awareness be enlarged to accommodate unpleasant realities that until now have existed only in secret.

Men seem to display the same symptoms as women victims—low self-esteem, depression, poor relationships, fear of intimacy, drug dependency and so on. But there may be one way in which an abused man's experi-ences differ from those of women: a strong sense of inadequacy and failure *as a man*. While women often find that they are regarded with suspicion if they are strong, men are seen as being beyond the pale if they show weakness or vulnerability. In our society, men are not sup-posed to be victims. They are expected to be able to look after them-selves, to resist, to fight back. These so-called masculine qualities are deeply rooted in our culture. They may be of dubious value, but all boys grow up in their shadow.

Many male survivors speak of anxiety about their sexual identity and orientation—not surprising when their central perception of 'what a man is' has been violated and distorted during childhood. These feelings of guilt, shame and failure seem to be shared equally by homosexual and heterosexual male survivors, and clearly make it harder for men to open up and start to talk about their problems. Male survivors can create elaborate strategies for survival as adults. They study, work hard, over-achieve, marry, raise children. But the abuse issue is often a time bomb, ticking silently away deep in their consciousness.

The stereotype of boy victims of sexual abuse is that they fall prey to rich gay pederasts, who seduce them with gifts and rides in sports cars and then involve them in drug-induced sexual orgies. The truth is very different. Most sexual abuse of boys, as of girls, takes place within the family. Another myth is that adolescent boys enjoy sexual experi-mentation with older men, and it does them no harm. Many male survivors talk of physical abuse in childhood, sometimes as part of sexual acts of masturbation or penetration, sometimes without any overt sexual activity.

Not surprisingly, it seems that men are still more reluctant than women to admit to having been abused. At ASCA we are contacted by far more women than men, a pattern consistent with reports from other countries. It is therefore particularly courageous of the men who have contributed to the book—and others who are facing their truth and all the pain it contains—to speak out.

To suggest that the incidence of abuse is higher for girls than for boys is curiously ignorant of the fact that—as women have been complaining for years—men are more reluctant to talk about their feelings. We just get angrier and perpetrate more overt, violent crimes ... the male way. But we won't talk about our pain because we're tough guys.

I'm a white heterosexual man. I've played a lot of sport, climbed the corporate ladder, done many masculine—even macho—things. I'm divorced with two teenage daughters. I was regularly beaten by both my parents until my early teens, and at the age of three was also sexually abused by a female babysitter. I emerged from childhood with deep emotional scars.

It took me a long time to find the courage to admit and acknowledge my vulnerability. I had to accommodate the fact that I had feelings at all! By controlling my feelings I'd crushed my passion, and in the process as an adult crushed the passion and expression of those around me. It was so hard to be honest about my emotions, and particularly about the anger and powerlessness associated with the abuse. I had to learn to release my anger in a controlled therapeutic environment, rather than on my family, subordinates at work and so on. Though I did not actually hit people, I did become controlling and manipulative. I felt I needed to control my environment to protect myself from the danger that I'd grown up to expect was always there. That was also part of the fear. If you're an abused male, you are both angry and afraid.

Taylor Shane

◆

For some, a process of recovering a traumatic memory of a past event precipitates a crisis. For others it's a more gradual wearing down of years of stubborn denial. This is how it was for me. For a long time I told myself that it didn't really happen ... well, not like that ... it wasn't meant that way. I accused myself of making a big deal out of nothing. Many of us reach middle age before the results of abusive events in childhood begin to surface. I was in my late forties when my doctor persuaded me to try group therapy sessions for survivors of abuse. We had to take turns to talk about our experiences. I felt embarrassed listening to some of the accounts because I thought I shouldn't really be there, that I had suffered very little in comparison with most of the other people in the group. Finally my turn came, and I read out a handwritten account of one abusive event in my childhood. I felt sure it was inadequate, and I couldn't look at any of them. When I finished there was total silence. Alarmed, I looked up. Their faces were frozen in horror, and two of the women were crying. That was the day I admitted to myself for the first time that I had suffered abuse as a child.

Until very recently, our culture generally approved of corporal punishment for children, especially boys. It toughened them up, taught them a quick lesson, prepared them for their role as men. The public tolerance of S&M societies and spanking clubs makes it harder to deny that there is often—maybe always—a sexual element when one human uses his power, status or authority to inflict pain on another. I always noticed at school that everyone was fascinated when someone got the strap or the cane. We'd try to watch, and always crowded around the victim afterwards to ask questions about it. When I discovered later in life that there were whole sections of pornographic bookstores devoted to men and women whipping and spanking each other, I felt very angry with that 'responsible' person who had so often taken advantage of me in childhood in this way for her own sexual pleasure.

Charles Andrews

✦

I was abused by an older male cousin when I was three years old. I was told that this was a secret; the secrecy of it all became deeply entrenched in my psyche. When I was ten I was raped by an older boy from a group I was hanging out with. Another boy held me down while he did it. I never told my mum about this as she didn't like that group of friends anyway, and I thought she'd get angry at me and think it was my fault.

I thought nothing more of it until I was about 12, when I went to high school and discovered the word 'poofter'. I used to wonder whether I was one of them. I decided I wasn't because I was attracted to girls. By the time I was 16 my friends were getting sexually active, but I was in no hurry. I've always been tall and looked older than I was, and between the ages of 14 and 18 I was approached by older women. I found this really scary, probably because the boys who raped me were older than me.

I fell in with a bunch of bikers when I was about 17, smoking dope, etc. I was still a virgin so I copped heaps from them. It was a bit in jest and a bit in nastiness; they were mainly ridiculing me. I didn't care really, except that for my eighteenth birthday they 'gave' me a girl. I didn't want to do it, but I had to or I would really have copped it from them. It was a horrible way to lose your virginity. I started dating girls regularly, though more for their company than for sex. I did have sexual relationships, though some of them turned out to be quite bizarre.

I was too trusting as a kid. Forgiveness is important to me, and in some ways I've forgiven my abusers, though I haven't forgotten what they did, and there are times when the hurt still comes flooding through.

David Cox

◆

FATHER, PLEASE
Father, please accept your son.
Say good things; things I need to know.
Don't tell me I'm not good enough.
Just be my Dad, and watch me grow.

Father, I just skinned my knee.
I know you told me not to run.
Don't yell and hit me, just because
I had to have a little fun.

Father, I fell off my bike.
My teeth are broken, please don't curse.
I'm scared and in such dreadful pain.
You work so hard to make it worse.

Dad, because I got it wrong,
Don't bash me till my arms are sore.
I cry. You say, 'That didn't hurt,'
And then you hit me even more.

Mother, please, I need your help.
Don't sit there while he pounds my arm,
And pulls my hair, and rants and swears.
Don't let him cause me all this harm.

Parents, please, don't fight it out.
Give me a hug or just a kiss.
Don't make me skim life's narrow surface.
It's no good having to live like this.

Dad, please say you love me. Just this once,
Allow these precious words to flow.
For I can't say them to my son,
And very soon he'll need to know.

Brian Bell

◆

The effects of abuse and the process of healing are probably much the same for men and for women. It is a lifetime's work, and it requires the trust and help of others. Contact with other men who'd travelled the road from emotional ignorance to emotional openness and freedom helped me a great deal. It was a revelation to discover other men who felt the same as I did. For a while they were my lifelines. Just knowing that I wasn't the only man having these difficulties was therapeutic for me. I found men who'd run huge corporations or their own businesses, doctors and lawyers, all in the same bind as myself.

Cecil Smith

Any perception that self-discovery is the domain of homosexual men is nonsense. I learned to cherish my sensitivity and strength and their most positive expressions. Finally, I discovered that persistence with therapy and trusting the process of self-discovery was most important. Eventually I realised that what I had suffered from had given me some of my greatest strengths. Through isolation and rejection I became strong and independent. Through being lied to, I learned to discern the truth and think for myself. Through being poor, I learned that happiness was not the result of possessions, of what you had, but of what you gave. Through living in fear of death, I learned what is really important in life— and that the need for love is greater than the fear of pain.

Joseph Elias

I have learned why I have been so angry, especially towards people in authority. Those in authority are not always unkind, and won't all want to sodomise me. It is clear that in some mixed-up way in the past I made such a connection, and I now understand where my anger, at times even violence, comes from. I offer no excuses for my behaviour, but search for the reasons that lie behind it. There is little doubt that my emotional development has been critically affected by those terrible and lonely years of my childhood.

Dave Owen

Sometimes people look back on their lives and wish they were different; I wanted to hide in the future. This kept me sane, kept me hoping, kept me alive. I could live in the illusions I created and not have to acknowledge my pain. For 30 long years I dragged my hurts and fears around with me, like a ball and chain—trying unsuccessfully to run from them. And when finally I could run no more, I realised I would never be able to escape who I was and find who I wanted to be, and I sat and cried and cried.

As an infant and repeatedly through my childhood years, men and women who were meant to be trustworthy and loving took advantage of me—sexually, physically and emotionally they repeatedly abused me. They derided and berated me, and used coercion to manipulate me until I agreed to do what they wanted. They repeatedly threatened that they would kill me if I ever told anyone what they did.

I could not escape them, I had nowhere to run—they were bigger, stronger, more powerful than I was. I hid where they could not reach me—in the farthest, darkest corner of my heart. I have remained there all this time, scared to death, always afraid that they would come back again just as they said they would. But although I hid there in order to survive, my life was no life at all—isolated in the dark dungeon of fear and pain and hate, I was empty and alone. I became my own enemy: in order to feel safe, I came to deny the life I so desperately wanted. I was never to reveal myself.

Emerging from this living death has been a huge struggle for me.

Joseph Elias

◆

I am married with three children, two sons and a daughter. At the age of 36, when I was working as an accounts manager, I began two years of therapy. My reason for seeking help was because of the effects of having been raped at the age of 14, and sexually assaulted over a two-year period by 11 different men. I had remained completely silent about these experiences. The effects were numerous, as were the difficulties associated with speaking out, which resulted in my losing my job. The attitudes towards abuse made many people in our dominant male culture regard my speaking out as unacceptable.

Paul Philips

◆

To write from the heart is to feel, and feeling is not something I normally do. The pain inside me is such a tremendous force that I do not have the courage or the strength to feel it. I'm so afraid of letting it go, because I don't know how big it is or when it would end. I'm so afraid of being let down that the risks of relying on anyone are too great. I'm so afraid of being hurt and used and laughed at and being tossed aside like a useless piece of garbage.

I feel as if I could cry and scream and tremble forever, and still not rid myself of all the turmoil that fills me. Why was I treated so meanly and abusively when I did nothing to deserve it? I was a happy, curious, inquisitive child. The adults who should have cared for me so easily broke through my childish defences. They forced me into a world that is not real, where I do not know how to act or what to do. The only defence I am left with is silence, and those who do not understand me reject me as being stupid or strange or unable to offer myself as a whole person. I can only shake my head and stare at the wall and wonder why I have been given so much to cope with when I only want to be loved and respected and cared about, as any person deserves to be. I can only hope that one day I will be able to lighten the load just enough to be able to have a rest and relax and enjoy some of the pleasures in life and start to see myself as a 'real' person, and not believe all the distorted images I have of myself as well as all the distortions I believe others see in me.

I never considered the fact that there might be others who feel the way I do. As I begin to meet and talk, through ASCA, with people who understand what I say and feel the same themselves, I find it that little bit easier to get through each day. I want to survive, and in doing so I want to help others survive and gain the courage and strength I'm beginning to find in myself. I want others to know there are people who care, and are thinking about them through all the hard times.

John T.

◆

ABUSE BY WOMEN

For a long time the idea of women abusers was regarded as preposterous. The truth is that while abuse by women may be less common than abuse by men, it is by no means rare. Emotional abuse by women is common-place; many women physically abuse children in the name of discipline or to vent their own rage; women also abuse sexually. Others fail to protect children by participating in abuse initiated by men, by colluding or by not intervening to prevent abuse. Of those who responded to a survey ASCA conducted, 36 per cent had been abused by women.

Women are capable of being just as self-serving, cruel, narcissistic, manipulative and criminal as men. The history of humanity is in part the oppression of the weak by the strong. Men prey on women and children, women prey on children (and occasionally men), and some of these children then persecute other children. From the evidence available to date, the majority of female offenders were abused themselves, and many of them offend in partnership (coerced or otherwise) with men. But this does not absolve them from responsibility for their actions, any more than male offenders are absolved.

Victims of abuse feel the same sense of devastation and betrayal whether their abuser is a man or a woman. But because society denies the fact that women abuse, survivors of female abusers experience particular difficulties when trying to accept their own truth about what was done to them. The disbelief these survivors encounter when they try to tell their story increases their sense of isolation, shame, confusion and guilt.

When we are children we are dependent on adults for food, shelter, cleanliness and comfort. We are in a physically intimate relationship with those who look after us, and particularly with our primary caregivers, who are most often women. When a caregiver crosses the boundaries and seeks sexual gratification and closeness from this necessary intimacy, or betrays it through violence and the use of physical power, the sense of betrayal is particularly devastating. This is true whether the child is a boy or a girl.

The child's difficulties are compounded if the abuser was their mother. The mother-child bond is regarded as the strongest, the most fundamental of any human relationship. Mother love has often been idealised, and, in a world run by men, motherhood has often been the only area of life where a woman has power. Abuse by our own mothers can cause the deepest wounds of all: 'If even my mother hurts me and does not love me, *I must be unlovable*'. These wounds can be the hardest of all to confront, the slowest of all to heal.

'Happy Mother's Day' they said on the radio. 'Happy Mother's Day' they said at the beginning of the church service. I bought a Sunday paper on the way home. It seems there was a competition to see who could bring Mother's Day into any article the most, from the TV guide to a well-known footballer cooking a roast chook for his mum for lunch, to another sports star ringing her mum on her mobile phone to tell her the good news about being selected for the Olympic team, to the sports or cooking or holidays sections, and of course all the ads for what you can get your mum for this 'wonderful day'.

Am I having a gripe? Yes. I am sick of the images of mums being such lovely creatures of warmth and love, security and safety. A mum who washes your clothes with such tenderness, or should be congratulated because she buys the right margarine. Some mothers might be like that, but my images are very different.

For the sake of the world she looked respectable, but in my eyes she was/is an evil, terrifying woman. You are supposed to be able to tell your mum when somebody hurts you, not see her getting her kicks while your dad rapes you.

There were some abuses she did in conjunction with others, and some she did on her own.

'No Mum, please don't lock me up again. Please can I have a teddy in there? Please let me out to go to the toilet, don't force me to make a mess.'

'Why do you have to scrub me so hard in the bath? I know I am dirty, but not many kids are dirty at three in the morning after their dad has taken them out. I know I mustn't make a sound, but it hurts so much.'

I'm angry. We live in a world that denies that mothers could be capable of hurting their own flesh and blood. Fathers, perhaps; but mothers? No way. Even some of the services designed to help incest victims shy away from abuse by mothers. Some feminists can't cope with the truth that members of their own sex would do these things.

As for me, have I sent a present of pink, fluffy slippers to my mum for today? Am I going to cook her roast chook for lunch? No. No. No.

She did teach me some worthwhile things in my childhood, but the ongoing legacy of her mothering is a hurt, bewildered, and angry woman.

I have strength. She did not teach me that strength, but I needed it to get through my childhood.

Next year on Mother's Day—weep. Weep for those of us who can't even weep for ourselves yet. And don't be blinded by the world's fantasy image of 'the mother'.

Jane Lewis

✦

Most abused people suffer from identity problems. To be aware that your mother sexually abused you when you were little results in a total loss of sexual identity. The overwhelming feeling is that you are different. To know that your mother used you for her own sexual gratification is completely and utterly devastating. I felt so different from everyone else at school. More recently, in support groups, I felt different from those who were abused by members of the opposite sex.

Jan Watson

◆

Recently I recovered memories of the abuse inflicted on me 60 years ago. It was a long, slow process that had started some 20 years earlier, when I was told that I had been adopted.

Gradually I pieced things together. I learned that I had been born in Scotland, that I had been in an institution for my first three years and that my birth mother was dead. In 1992 I visited Scotland, and met some people who had known my natural mother. I was given her wedding ring and watch, and returned home believing that I had come to terms with my past. Not so!

Over the next few months I became more unsettled and angry. I returned to the counsellor I had seen a couple of years earlier about my feelings of anger. During one session I related an anecdote my adoptive father had told me about myself when I was little, and referred to someone he said had been my kindergarten teacher. At my counsellor's suggestion, I went home and concentrated on what I could remember of this person.

I put on a tape of gentle music, sat down and wrote the woman's name in the centre of a sheet of paper. Then I wrote around the name all the words that my mind associated with her. As I did this I was surprised to find that I was getting a strong genital response. Later I drew a picture of the woman and myself. It was quite extraordinary. The words described violence, sex and misery; the picture represented a tiny child's terror. At first I didn't want to believe that I had been the victim of physical and sexual abuse, but gradually I remembered more details.

The woman was the supervisor of the institution where I lived, which trained nurses in mothercraft. She was my principal carer and had a great deal of power. Her behaviour to me alternated between violence and expressions of love associated with sexual abuse.

At last I understood my behaviour throughout my life. My self-control, my lack of feelings, my difficulties with sex, my fantasies that sex and violence belong together, all fell into place. I had 'forgotten' the abuse in order to survive, and like so many others, survive I have.

I found it very difficult to grasp the concept of a woman as abuser, as do those I have told, because our society sees women as carers. With all the publicity about paedophilia concentrating on male perpetrators, I feel like an aberration, but I would like my story to be told.

Jean McKendrick

◆

I hesitate to write this story as it brings back so many painful memories. I was born in Canton, China in 1936. An ugly baby girl, I was a big disappointment to my mother. It was a difficult birth, and in those days medical facilities were limited—I was later told I had endangered my mother's life.

My mother rejected me, and my grandmother came out from the village to look after me. I was sent to the village to stay with her until I was about three years old. When I returned to Canton to live with my parents and sister I was very unhappy. At night I used to wet the family bed (we all slept together). My mother would get furious, and for punishment I was beaten with a leather strap.

Our family came to Australia when I was ten. We lived in a flat above my father's grocery business. During this time I was often beaten. My younger sister, who my mother loved, would pick fights with me when we were playing; my mother always sided with her, and called me hurtful names while hitting me with the cane end of the feather duster. I remember frequently going to school with welts on my legs.

When I was 15 my mother made me stop going to school and begin work. We weren't badly off, but she wanted me to earn money. I didn't speak English well and couldn't write much, so I enrolled in evening school. I spent a lot of time at night studying, but my mother resented my nights at school as by then she had four more children and wanted more help at home. She began accusing me of going out with boys at night rather than studying. There was a lot of tension at home and I was constantly being harassed. I subsequently had a breakdown because of working, studying and all the trouble at home. I cried all the time, and couldn't eat or sleep.

I decided to get away, but in those days girls didn't leave home until they got married. By the time I was 22 I had saved enough money to be able to buy a house with one of my brothers, but my mother refused me permission to do this. She forced me to buy a car instead, which would help her run the business.

Shortly before my father died he called my mother and me together and told us that he wanted to leave his half share of the business to me to repay me for all I had done for them. My mother was angry, insisted that it wasn't necessary and that she wanted the whole business in her name. Because my father was a sick man I didn't want to see them quarrelling. I told him not to worry about it, and let Mum have the business. Now I wish I hadn't.

A few years ago I raised the matter of the past, of how I had been abused and exploited. My mother's response was to start a rumour that I had gone crazy. Some of my sisters and a brother told me that Mum had said they were not to speak to me as I am insane.

There is nothing I can do about her and the past. Thank God

I have three lovely children who are all doing well, and a husband who supports me.

Choy Sue Aung

◆

A SONG OF CHILDHOOD
'Jah-ni-iss!' a loud screech interrupts me.
'Jah-ni-iss!
Where is that dratted girl?
Never there when you want her.
Why am I so unlucky?
The ugliest girl in the world—
Jah-ni-iss!'

Oh no. I'm found,
Dragged by my ear or hair.
The song of my childhood continues:
'Why am I so unlucky?
You never think about me.
What will my friends think?
What will the neighbours think?
Nobody likes you, you're so ugly.
Nobody likes you, you're such a nuisance.'

I never reply, but stand still waiting.
Here it comes—the stick, strap, wooden spoon or hand,
The daily beatings.
The song continues:
'It's good for your character, you wicked girl.
Why am I so unlucky?'

Always told I'm ugly, my voice is awful,
Just looking at me makes them sick.
My fed-up mother and I try to kill me,

I want to return to the spirits.
Father rescues me every time.

I try to escape into marriage.
Oh no, three new torturers added on.
Rape, too, is added to improve me.
I'm divorced years later.

Mother's song continues.
At forty I laugh, and tell her she's fired as mother—
I am finally in charge of me.
Defeated, she leaves with shoulders bowed.
Suddenly she looks old,
While I have grown up,
An adult at last.

Janice

◆

Mother's Day 1996 brings flashes of Mother's Day many years ago, when I was eight years old. My siblings and I queued up in the morning to shake our mother's hand and recite the verses we had learned. My part was, *'Meiner Mutter Hande sind von der Arbeit schwer, dennoch streicheln sic so lind wie sonst keine mehr.'* Roughly translated, this says, 'My mother's hands are heavy from work, yet they stroke me with an unsurpassed gentleness.'

It was a lie. It was all a lie! There was no way in the world I could say these words. Everyone looked at me while I pressed my lips shut. I was not going to say it. Her hands did not stroke; her hands hit, poked, probed, pinched, pressed, pulled, squeezed—hers were hands that hurt.

I looked at her. She had tears in her eyes as she proudly observed her many sons and daughters lining up to wish her 'Happy

Mother's Day'. Tears in her eyes—more lies! Memories of cold, cold eyes looming over me. Goose bumps when I realised what would come next. Cold eyes.

Our cult had approximately 100 members, and about 40 of these were women.

I am at a friend's house. She is my closest friend. Hesitatingly I speak about the excruciating pain of having to come to terms with the fact that not only did my mother not protect me, she actively abused me. My friend's immediate response was, 'Your mother was a victim too'.

I withdraw. I am confused. Does this mean that as a victim I should feel compassion for my abuser? I am in so much pain. Does my friend ask me to put this aside and consider the pain my abuser must have been in? And what about me as a child abused by my mother? Does the fact that my abuser was also a victim mean that the pain she inflicted was less severe? How cruel people can be in their denial.

I love women. I love our bodies. I love having sex with women. I love a woman's softness, her sense of humour, the way a woman sees the world. I prefer the company of women. Women inspire me and make me happy. Despite my having been abused by women, many women, sexually, emotionally, physically. Cruel women. Cold women. Hateful women. Evil women. Ordinary women. Because I love women I will not be silenced about the abuse women inflict.

Phoenix Van Dyke

◆

To be abused shatters one's soul. To be abused by your own sex, a mother figure, carries the betrayal to an even deeper part of you. For me, the abuse by my adopted mother had profound long-term effects.

Her sexual abuse of me was not the only betrayal. She failed to protect me from a male sexual abuser, a so-called family friend.

She betrayed me to a life of violence in an alcoholic home. It was hell. All this from a woman who according to society's ideal (and mine) was supposed to love, protect and nurture me into my own beautiful potential. How did I respond? I was dumbfounded! I withdrew into a world of make-believe and dissociation. To cope, I would immerse myself in hyperactivity—sport, study, cleaning, perfectionism; and humour was a constant shield. Who would guess that the school clown was being sexually abused? Behind this confident, jovial face lay such immeasurable suffering. The mask was what I needed to maintain my fantasy. I planned one day to escape—and at 16 I ran away. The last laugh was mine!

So why did the betrayal by a woman have such devastating implications? It meant the loss of a mum, and this left a horrible aching void that stayed with me till I was 33 years old. For so long I searched in every female face for a potential 'mum', someone who would love me. I longed to be held in tender arms, and not to be abused but to feel safe and secure. Only then could I mature naturally, as I was meant to do. Also, I felt that my adopted mum had great powers. Her threats bound me in fear—it was as if she had a hold on me, she was inside my mind. I didn't want to believe that this woman was abusing me, because she was all I had then, so I maintained a fantasy that she was 'ideal'.

My recovery meant finding a healthy, natural way to fill the void within me. I needed to be nurtured into maturity. I would go to older trusted female friends for long hugs, though first I had to restore my trust and desensitise myself to touch. My counsellor would work session after session to help me get used to safe touch again, to help me learn that touch does not always mean abuse. Before she helped me, if someone touched me even in a kind and gentle way, my skin would feel as if it was burning. Eventually, I learned how nice it is to be cuddled. Then, little by little, I was able to let go of my searching for a mum, and began to fill up on the inside.

For a long while I saw myself as sexless, genderless. I did not like my own body until, in my thirties, I began adolescence. Ha! As part of my recovery I began to take pride in my appearance, and experimented till I found the 'right fit' for me. I was going to live my life my way. I had a war cry: 'I'm not going to let the bastards beat me!' Instead, I'm going to do all that they said I could never do, and more, just to spite them, just to love myself!

Anna Foster

◆

At the age of four, on several occasions during cult ceremonies, I was sexually abused and tortured by women, having already been abused by my uncle since I was a baby. Being raped and tortured by either sex is extremely painful, being raped by someone of my own sex left me feeling more confused. I couldn't understand why someone without a penis would want to penetrate me. I now understand that the women were out to gain power by using my body. Their behaviour was no different from the men's—they were just as evil and abusive.

Being abused by women affected all my relationships with other females. This included my mother, relatives, teachers and friends. I felt distant from all of them. I hated being touched, was afraid of being touched. I didn't know why, as I'd blocked the abuse from my memory. It also affected my feelings towards my body, which I hated. I hated being a girl, I didn't want to have a vulva or breasts. During my teenage years I'd physically feel fear and tension or numbness. This didn't change much until after I'd remembered that I was abused.

It took a long time, and a lot of help, for me to look at women while staying aware of my own body. It is still difficult to do; I have reclaimed most of my body, but some parts remind me of the abusers, and even now seem to belong to them rather than to me.

Skyy Bright

◆

Surviving abuse by women; surviving abuse by men: how is it different?

I was in a 'family of origin' therapy group in the days when I still thought of myself as an incest survivor: no major ritual abuse memories had yet surfaced, and I was even farther away from recognising myself as someone with multiple personalities. The therapist asked us to draw a picture of the power relations in our family, using different shapes, sizes and colours for each child and each parent. My father was a large red rectangle, much bigger than any of the children, but my mother was an absolutely enormous blue dome, arching over everybody, my father included.

It had been clear to me for some time that whatever my issues with my father, my issues with my mother were much bigger. Here was an unmistakable graphic representation of that truth. The therapist asked me what gave my mother so much power. At the time I—the 'I' then at the front of my personality system—did not know.

My conscious mind registered my mother as a pillar of the community, an elder of the church, who was respected by teachers and neighbours as a good Samaritan and always did the right thing. She was a bit of a martyr to my father's moods and demands, a good housewife, and a charming hostess to his business friends. She very seldom lost her cool, but when she did, by God it was time to run for cover.

No one asked how or why there was such a deep and abiding rage hidden inside this woman. She hit me more often than the other children, my older sister tells me, and often for things that were clearly not my fault. And she certainly had no idea of how to protect her daughters. When I complained, at about the age of six, because her uncle would make me sit on his lap while he fondled and kissed me, she said the least I could do was to let a lonely old man cuddle me. When I was distressed, at the age of 12, because I had been talked into sitting down next to some bloke while I was walking the dog at the beach, and had subsequently been touched up, she said he was probably just a lonely man looking for love. It didn't seem to worry her that he'd only let me go when I'd promised to return that night; I suppose I should be grateful that she didn't expect me to keep the promise!

If I was in pain, I was told I was dramatising, making a fuss about nothing. Once my little finger got caught in somebody's car door. The finger was nearly off, but she didn't take me to the doctor. She bound it up herself and then told me to stop making such a fuss or she'd give me something to cry about.

Because of my own experiences, I am impatient with feminist arguments that the dominance of men, our patriarchal society, is the root of all evil. Certainly I am all for challenging male attitudes, and laws and practices that demean or subjugate women. But we need to challenge women's misuse of power as well.

Miriam Wainwright

◆

I believe such a thing as emotional sexual abuse exists. This belief is based on my experiences with my mother, and how utterly dirty and violated I felt at the time. One of her favourite names for me was 'tunnel-cunted slut'. She used to sneer, 'You've had every man and his dog up you'; 'Dirty whore, you'd fuck anything'. I endured things like this right through my teens.

She used to throw me out of the house and tell me she hoped I would get raped. When she found out I had been, she'd say things like, 'You enjoyed it, didn't you? You really raped him, didn't you?'

Sexual abuse is not just physical; it can be verbal too. For many years I couldn't see that. She was my mother, and mothers don't sexually abuse. Yet I accept now that she did violate me. And I comfort and value that confused young girl inside me. I no longer believe the lies she told me about myself. What I still struggle to deal with is the pain arising from the fact that her abuse was interspersed with the occasional kindness. This makes her abuse more insidious. I don't see her any longer—a necessary move for my stability.

Louise Plummer

✦

SADISTIC ABUSE

There is no single definition of sadistic abuse. While some may label their abuse sadistic only if it was very extreme, many people define it on the basis of the perpetrator's intentions rather than on his or her actions. People who define their abuse in this way may see it as torture rather than abuse. Sadistic abuse may be emotional, sexual or physical, or it may be too bizarre to fit into any of these categories. For example, while an act may gratify the perpetrator sexually it may not conform to what people would generally regard as sexual behaviour. Sadistic abuse may include any especially cruel abuse; it may be a single incident or may continue for years.

The motivation of sadistic and non-sadistic perpetrators is different, and their behaviour can traumatise victims differently. Non-sadistic perpetrators often establish an environment in which they can convince themselves that the victim has consented and is enjoying the abuse, or that the abuse is for the victim's own good. They ignore the victim's own feelings altogether. Sadistic perpetrators, on the other hand, do not ignore the victim's pain. Their infliction of pain is intentional rather than being a consequence of their actions. Their own pleasure is directly linked to how much the victim suffers, so they pay close attention to maximising the victim's suffering and therefore their own enjoyment.

The specific problems survivors of sadistic abuse face are likely to include a terror of showing emotion; feeling worse rather than better after showing emotion in any way; lack of any feelings at all; 'paranoid' symptoms; feelings of being evil, hideous, not even human; an inability to fit into general survivor groups or find self-help books helpful; extreme dissociative symptoms; and a belief that the world is malevolent. We hope that the courage of the contributors who have written about their abuse will enable readers to clarify whether their own abuse was sadistic, and help them to understand some of the symptoms they experience.

I am a survivor of sadistic abuse, which was inflicted on me by both my parents. I remember very little of my life. Apart from a few incidents of specific extreme abuse, the rest is too hazy to describe. My memories started to return before I entered therapy, and I found them very hard to reconcile with the fact that my parents were also caring, responsible people with a good sense of humour and a great deal of generosity. I did always remember that as a child I had thought I had two sets of parents: one good, one evil.

When I read material written by incest survivors I am often surprised that they are encouraged to tell their abusers, 'I was really hurt by you and I want you to know it'. Even as an adult the last thing I would want is to give them the satisfaction of knowing how much they hurt me. The implications of this are played out when my therapist wants me to show my distress at the abuse I suffered. Logically I know her intentions are good, but emotionally I feel she too is abusive. It seems that all she wants to do is make me cry, and that makes me suspicious. For me, crying is nearly impossible and if I do cry I often feel worse, not better. It can make me feel terrified and ashamed. I also assumed that my therapist wanted me to describe the details of the abuse because while she pretended it was disgusting, she actually found it a turn-on. There was no way to find out what she really thought. I had become so accustomed to compulsive liars I couldn't trust anyone.

I used to berate myself about the fact that support/therapy groups for incest survivors didn't seem to help me. I thought the reason I felt like a freak was because I just wasn't trying hard enough to fit in. And I found that once I disclosed to people, any positive feelings I had for them turned to hatred. I then felt unsafe and couldn't go back. I also felt I couldn't tell others my story because it would make them pity me or they would use it to aid their own denial (by thinking they had no right to complain because someone else's life was worse). But now I attend a self-help group for people with dissociative identity disorder, and I don't feel my story is unusual there.

Sadistic abuse places the child in a double bind. If I show I am hurt he/she/they will delight in my pain, and their perverse pleasure will encourage me to believe I have brought further degradation on myself. If I pretend I haven't been hurt I may save myself this humiliation, but it will encourage them to try harder, to increase the abuse until they know they have achieved the satisfaction of breaking me. Whichever option I choose will hurt me more. There's no way out. And because the choice is mine, whatever happens is my fault.

It took me a long time to understand that this was why I couldn't express anger. From books, groups, etc. on healing all I found was that survivors have difficulty with anger as they can be scared of not releasing it constructively, or of being overpowered by it. I am yet to read about my problem with anger, which is that to show it is to allow abusers to get off on it. I don't know how to overcome the feeling that expressing anger (to anyone) is to set myself up for abuse. My abusers took from me even that option for empowerment. Disclosure for me doesn't bring relief, it brings terror.

It was the safest option in childhood not to express any emotion at all. These blocks have stayed in place, and make intimacy nearly impossible. The choice is agonising. Either I meet my need for safety by not connecting with people and remain lonely, or I meet my need for intimacy by opening up and then suffer the terror of this lack of safety. It has taken me years to establish even the most basic level of trust. The self-hatred associated with disclosure has made the changes taking place in therapy seem like a deterioration rather than an improvement. The lack of trust this demonstrates can appear very paranoid indeed. But now I am beginning to see things more clearly, and have the capacity to be honest with myself and others. I thought my history would leave me with a permanent legacy of dislike (even terror) of human beings, but happily that has started to shift. I no longer see myself as indescribably bad.

It also took me a long time to realise that many of my problems were related to the abuse. I thought I could talk to a counsellor about the incest, but that I would need a psychiatrist to help me with the 'schizophrenic' symptoms. I didn't know these symptoms were dissociative mechanisms that had helped me cope with the abuse. Therapy was the hardest thing I have ever done. I even seriously thought my therapist might have been employed by my parents to find out if I would disclose, and that when I did I would be declared insane.

The most rewarding thing I have learned is to take responsibility for my own life. I used to think, 'They ruined my life, why should I be lumbered with the responsibility of fixing it?' Because I had not been taught how to take care of myself or take responsibility for myself I wasted time hoping others would fix my problems. I even retraumatised myself by maintaining contact with my family (who claim I have 'false memories') and thinking they had changed just because I wanted them to.

I don't want conflict in my life, and I couldn't resolve the conflict unless I forgave them. But how can you forgive someone who is not sorry? That's not forgiveness, that's denial. Removing my family from my life was no easy thing, but it was the first step in taking control of my life and becoming the person I want to be. Since then I have felt empowered to make other big changes and not continue procrastinating out of fear.

While I cannot change my past, I can choose to transform the present and the future into something better.

Veronica Taylor

◆

My family environment was so violent it was like living in a concentration camp. Conflict and chaos was the norm. The atmosphere was horrendous: my parents yelled and screamed at each other constantly, and daily life consisted almost entirely of fights and squabbling.

My father was very cruel and sadistic, and it was really dangerous because you never knew when he was going to fly into a rage and threaten to kill you. I remember how he would drag me by the hair or throw me out of bed to make me get ready for school. I was often thrown across a room, beaten with sticks, dog leads or belts, and had things thrown at me. I was slapped around the face and head if he was in a bad mood. Unfortunately he was often like this. He had so much anger, hatred and rage inside him.

My father used to derive pleasure from seeing me afraid. He used to back me against the wall with glee, and I can still see the satisfied look on his face and the power he felt by seeing the fear in my eyes. That look was hideous, and I made a point of trying not to give him the pleasure of seeing me afraid. It was the only way I could fight back, so I learned to numb out and dissociate from all my feelings. I was very sensitive, and this was the only way I could cope.

I was deeply hurt that my mother just allowed it to go on, and pretended it wasn't happening. I always think of her being like an ostrich, burying her head in the sand and hoping that the problem would go away. I feel the abuse I received from my mother was that she would deny my reality or make excuses for my father's behaviour. Not being validated for the pain I suffered or being protected in any way has also contributed to my denial of my feelings.

As an adult I also used to minimise what had happened to me, and tell myself that it didn't really affect me. But I did remember a lot of the sadistic abuse and violence, whereas my sister and younger brother haven't—they have blocked it all out.

Since working on healing my childhood pain I have come to understand some of the things my parents went through themselves that resulted in their behaviour towards me. My family history is full of hiding, covering up and secrecy. I understand now how things are passed on from generation to generation, and how the pattern of abuse is often repeated. I am determined to break the cycle, to heal my childhood wounds and change the negative behaviour patterns that I adopted because of my abuse. I am happy to say that it really is worth it: my life is improving so much.

Linda Honey

♦

It still feels difficult at times to think about the grossly sadistic things I experienced as a child. I remember what it was like to feel as though I was the only person in the world who had experienced such horror, and that nobody would understand. Even now I feel an urge to protect people from the facts. My hope is that, through writing, I can help others who have experienced sadistic abuse to feel less isolated.

When I was a child of nine or ten the family friend who was sexually abusing me also made me available, on two occasions, to other men. I was raped, urinated upon and otherwise tortured by groups of adult males, including being burned with cigarettes on the soles of my feet. I suppose they must have been some sort of organised paedophile group. Very little seems to be known or understood about groups of people who abuse children, and I find the scarcity of available information disappointing.

These people thrive on secrecy. They must be exposed. I registered one perpetrator's name with the police through Operation Paradox. That's perhaps the best I can do without compromising my own safety. It does make me very angry sometimes.

My experiences caused me to wonder if I'd ever feel clean again. I wanted to die. I'd like to tell anybody who has had a similar experience that living with it, healing and a restored sense of innocence and dignity are possible. I can now bear to think of the disgusting things done to me, and I love me, I love that child they tortured. I am determined to do whatever I can to challenge the activities of these people who ruin other people's childhoods with their cruelty.

Louise Plummer

◆

I always knew my mother was a monster, I just never knew why. I didn't realise that what I went through was different from other people's experiences. I thought all mothers were like mine. It was no shock to me that I was abused, it was all I knew—but I was shocked that not everyone is abused. Even now I still see it this way.

My mother was a twisted sadistic bitch. You could see it in her eyes. Something would flick a switch in her, and suddenly the threat of losing my life would be very real. Her attitude to me was, 'I hate your fucking guts and I'd like to kill you but I can't because I need someone to do the housework'. My shrink says she was psychotic as she had no empathy, and even bad parents usually have some empathy. She detested me crying, and it would trigger her to be even more sadistic.

To maintain secrecy and compliance some incest survivors I know were threatened with being put in a home or something like that. My mother never made such idle threats. She would just threaten to kill me, and because of her behaviour I had no reason to doubt that she meant it.

One issue I struggle with is understanding her intentions. How much did she know and plan, and how much did she just chance upon the outcomes? Did she know mind control techniques? Everything she did served to annihilate me and was part of some family conspiracy. She would attack me in front of them, and yet they would say I was lucky to have such a 'wonderful mother'. This served to kill off any faint hope I had that anyone would ever help me. She even claimed to know what I was thinking, and would hit me until I confessed my thoughts. Then she would then hit me again for thinking them. So I learned that even thinking my own thoughts was dangerous.

Emotional sadism does more damage than physical—like being told, 'I can kill you whenever I like', or 'I gave you life and I can take it away again'. Sadistic abuse is the death of hope. It wasn't as though she was angry and became abusive, what she did was just part of who she was. I felt like an insect being experimented on to see how much it could take.

One difficult aspect of sadistic abuse is that it forces you to confront and accept the sadistic side of yourself. This is especially true if you're someone with multiple personalities, as you'll probably have parts identical to the abuser. I had to acknowledge that I'm capable of doing the same things as her, but the important difference is that I choose not to. I can see how everyone is capable of sadism. I also felt nothing but murderous rage towards children. 'Ordinary' incest survivors probably don't suffer from a child-phobia so bad that it makes you get up and leave whenever a baby is nearby.

While some survivors of sadistic sexual abuse say they don't have feelings of guilt about the abuse because it was never even remotely pleasurable, I did feel guilty. I thought that because I had the choice between participating or being killed, if I didn't really want the sexual abuse I would have let her kill me instead.

Information about concentration camps kept me alive. The Nazis assumed you weren't human, and it was totally random when they picked on you. In the camps you didn't know whether or not you would die today, and if you did it wouldn't matter to anyone. This was just like my mother. It kept me going, as I realised that the shit she inflicted on me was not personal.

One result of her treatment of me that I have found difficult to overcome is that I never leaned how to say or do anything nice to anybody. I could never say anything genuinely positive to anyone, though I faked it well enough to maintain jobs, relationships, etc.

The way I learned to be genuinely kind was through having cats! If you say something nice to a person it makes you vulnerable, and they'll get the upper hand, but with cats it's not so dangerous. It was only after I had learned to be nice to cats that I was able to try it out on humans too.

Louise Baptista

◆

I was abused by my uncle, a sadist and satanist. The abuse I endured was extremely painful physically and emotionally. My uncle would usually torture me by attacking my genitals with sharp objects before or while raping me. He would always make out that I was being punished—that is, that he was torturing me because I didn't want to be sexually active. I was four years old. To add to the intense pain I suffered because of his sadistic deeds at home, he also took me along to cult ceremonies. Here I was stuck with a group of psychopathic, satanic sadists, all out to sexually, physically and mentally rape and torture me. This is the extreme end of sadism: they seemed to thrive on the sight of me and other children suffering.

Fortunately I survived. Many didn't. As a result of my harrowing childhood I grew up feeling numb, very tense, and constantly afraid of being punished. I never knew why I felt this way because I'd blocked out all the abuse from my memory. I lived in fear and always remained alert, ready to run if someone was to attack me in some way. I was 21 when I remembered that my uncle had raped and tortured me. From then on I began to understand where my fears about people disliking and hurting me came from. I spent a few hundred hours in therapy and a lot more time on my own working on healing.

In time I was able to stand in my front yard without fearing that I was going to be hurt or killed, though I still can't stand out there on my own for long. My fears of being punished have eased a great deal. I am able to talk to strangers with a smile and know

I'm usually safe. I feel alone, lonely and unlovable at times, but have come far enough in my healing journey to know that most people are not evil and are not out to hurt me or other people.

Skyy Bright

◆

RITUAL ABUSE

Ritual abuse is defined as the brutal and systematic abuse of children, adolescents or adults, consisting of physical, sexual, psychological and spiritual abuse and involving the use of rituals. It is usually carried out by multiple perpetrators in the name of an ideology, and often involves repeated abuse over an extended period of time.

Ritual abuse aims at gaining ultimate control over another human being. This control is attempted through torture of the mind, body and spirit. The abusive practices are often handed down from generation to generation, and the principal victims are small children. Many groups that perpetrate ritual abuse are also involved in making and distributing child pornography, in child prostitution and other forms of organised crime.

Ritual abuse is also known as satanic ritual abuse and organised sadistic abuse. Many people have been abused within a satanic belief system, though abuse also takes place in the name of other ideologies and deities. The worshipped deity is usually a destructive one.

The main tool perpetrators of ritual abuse use to maintain control over their victims is a child's ability to dissociate from the reality of the abuse. Children who can dissociate well make good victims. A child who can continue to live a 'normal' life while at the same time suffering horrendous abuse that they are able to 'forget' is easily controlled. Many people who have suffered ritual abuse have developed dissociative identities (also known as multiple personalities) as a defence mechanism against the abuse.

In 1992 Australian survivors of ritual abuse started speaking out publicly about the crimes perpetrated against them, and got together to form Ritual Abuse Survivors and Supporters (RASS), with offices in three states. A few months later the first issue of *Beyond Survival*, a bi-monthly magazine on ritual abuse, trauma and dissociation, was published. At the same time, professionals working with ritual abuse survivors began to work towards establishing greater awareness of this crime. They formed the Australian Association of Trauma and Dissociation, whose annual conference is attended by professionals from all over Australia and New Zealand.

Statistics kept by sexual assault services in Canberra showed that during two sample weeks in 1995 they were contacted by more women stating that they had been ritually abused than by rape victims. The Sydney Rape Crisis Center received 584 calls between July 1994 and June 1995 from women who identified themselves as ritual abuse survivors.

Ritual abuse survivors have been speaking out for a long time, but it is only in the last few years that some people have become willing to listen. Those of you who have not been affected by ritual abuse will find it very difficult to believe these stories—as we did. The abuse is so horrific that it seems impossible it could have happened here in Australia. But perhaps after the recent surfacing of 'unbelievable' cases overseas, such as the Fred and Rosemary West case in England or the Marc Dutroux case in Belgium, more people may begin to listen.

It is very difficult for such survivors, who are not believed, and who are specifically excluded from government help in some states. When ritual abuse perpetrators in Australia are taken to court the survivor's lawyer usually recommends that the ritual elements of the abuse be left out to avoid damaging the credibility of the victim. Nevertheless, some brave people, including children, have been speaking out.

I had a terrible father. He did bad things when I went to his house every Friday. At night, when I was fast asleep, he would wake me up and say, 'We are going somewhere'. Then he would put me into his car in my pyjamas and take me to a place that was shaped like a wide cement tunnel. The tunnel was near the seaside. When we were inside, I saw men in black capes and clothes and women in black as well. When they saw my father they said, 'Now let us pray to Satan'. They said kind things about the devil. When that was over, they had little baby bunnies that were very sweet and I got to pat them and hug them and give them names. Then they snatched them off me and when I was trying to shut my eyes and think about something else, they chopped their heads off.

One night we went to a forest. The same people were there. The forest was very dark except for candles. There was an upside-down cross. They made a child who was there take his clothes off and then they took photos and a video of him. He was trying not to do the things they said, but they made him walk up and down. They had a whip. They did all the rude things to me too. They took photos and videos of me. The women and the men touched my private parts.

I was desperate to tell Mummy about what happened. I told her and Nanny. Some police came to hear the story. I was really happy when it was all over. When we went to court I tried to speak up, but I was very scared and embarrassed. The person I was with took me outside to get a drink and a little walk. I was too scared to go back. My sister spoke up and that is the reason he went to jail for a while.

It frightens me a lot. I see demons sometimes. Often I nearly faint. I am scared that one day the court will be on his side and we will have to go and see him again.

I don't think I am very much like the other children at school. They all have good families. They have nice fathers and I wish we had one as well. I will be afraid of him all my life.

I wished I was dead when they killed the poor rabbits. I saw some people killed too, but I don't really like talking about that.

I love God and wish that there was no such thing as the devil. Sometimes I see my guardian angel at the side of my bed and I think the angels are guarding me to keep the devil away. When I go to see Dr A., it makes me feel that the devil is going further down every time we go there. Dr A. writes down the things and has special rubbers that she rubs out my bad memories with.

Robert Somerville, aged 8

◆

I didn't realise anything was wrong till I was about three years old. Then I did not want to be alive any more because of the terrible things that were happening.

The person doing most of the rude things was my father. There were other people in this too. Some of them were women and some were men. There were other children who were having the same things done to them as me. The bad people took rude videos and photos of us. My brother was there too. Mummy was at home and did not know what was happening to us.

The bad people dressed up and there were things done to animals. What happened to the rabbits was that they got killed for a sacrifice. Also they killed children too. I told the police about two women my brother and I saw stabbed to death.

I tried to tell Mummy when I was three but I couldn't. When I was six I told Mummy about the bad things that were happening. I thought she would smack me and tell me that I was lying. I was so scared, because the bad people said if I told anyone they would kill me.

When I told the police I felt a bit embarrassed. When I went to court I felt even more embarrassed about telling so many people and also having my father there. Anyway I told the court and he was sent to jail for a while, but got out.

I do not think of it very much. Sometimes I do have bad dreams about it. I am still angry with all the bad people for doing those things. I feel safe now, because the bad people can't find us where we live, but if they did find us they would probably do more bad things to us.

> You should never trust anyone, even your own parents.
>
> *Sarah Somerville, aged 9*

◆

I am a survivor of early childhood sexual and satanic ritual abuse. I endured being repeatedly raped and systematically tortured by my uncle and his friends. I was told during the abuse that the female abusers were my mothers and that there was no safety for me anywhere. I also was forced to participate in cannibalism.

I completely blocked out all the abuse in order to survive, and it remained blocked out for 16 years. During these years I lived a miserable life. I felt I was unlovable, worthless, ugly and putrid inside. I found it difficult to talk to most people, including my peers, teachers, relatives and my immediate family. Being with a lot of people left me wishing that I'd disappear forever or die. When I was asked a question in class, I'd be silent or give a quick and quiet answer and put my head down, hoping the teacher would go on to the next student.

I'd have a panic attack each time I saw a dog, even if it was on the other side of a park, because I had been raped by one. As I was growing up I couldn't have survived if I had had any conscious knowledge of the abuse I endured. I didn't have the strength, skills or support to deal with the horrors of my childhood. My life was filled with fear and anguish. I believe that if I'd remembered as a child or teenager, it would have killed me.

During my late teens, my mental and emotional health deteriorated a great deal, yet I managed to pass Year Twelve and go to university. After two years I could no longer bear the strains of studying and being surrounded by groups of people and I dropped out. I was fortunate to find a brilliant therapist. He was caring, understanding, wise and always had my best interests at heart. As I learned to trust him and for the first time felt heard and loved, I began to remember. Initially I'd faint in many of our therapy sessions. I found it hard to move, walk, talk, eat good food, socialise, read, write, shop or watch television. My life was turned upside down. All my energy and resources were sucked up by the awareness of my uncle betraying me, a man I had believed loved me. I worked on my healing every day. I didn't have the emotional or mental space to study, go to work, party, attend family functions—my life was just about healing.

I still have a long way to go before I completely recover from my harrowing childhood. I am halfway up the mountain that I've been climbing for years, and I'm looking forward to reaching the top.

Skyy Bright

◆

My first major breakthrough in consciously dealing with the reality of severe abuse throughout my infancy, childhood and teenage years came when I recognised and named myself as a survivor of incest. Until then, if you had asked me about my family of origin, I would have described it as better than average.

The closeness between us—between me and my sisters, between me and each of my parents, between me and my brother—seemed rare. It was real enough, but now I see it as the kind of intimacy that comes from shared terror, shared subjection to torture and brainwashing, shared reliance on maintaining amnesiac barriers between the parts of our personalities that knew the truth, and the parts that needed to be able to function in the day-to-day world— parts that went to school, passed exams, looked good in interviews, performed in jobs, survived.

The things that look so good came from the things that were indescribably, unbelievably bad. My youngest sister, a publisher, has attributed her career and her success to my reading aloud to her and to my other younger sister throughout childhood. I read aloud to both my sisters, and the elder of them read aloud to the youngest when she woke in terror from nightmares in the middle of the night. My main avenue was books. I would read anything,

anything to escape. As we grew up we each read books for ourselves. In my early teens I was at times reading three books a day, emerging only briefly and reluctantly into daily reality to eat meals or say hallo or goodbye at social gatherings.

It took me a year of damned hard work to break through to the ritual abuse memories. I really, really thought I was 'just' working on incest. I had body memories of a hand squeezing my throat; afterwards my throat felt bruised. I knew that force had been used on me. I knew I had been raped. But why, why, when I tried to go farther, would I keep running into this wall, this black wall of utter terror? How much worse could it have been? What more could they have done? Surely there were limits?

I have found, to my cost, that there are virtually no limits.

How can I blame my family for not facing the reality of ritual abuse, when I know how hard it has been for me to fight the programming and to deal constructively with my own overwhelming rage, terror and grief? Just staying alive, let alone staying sane, has been a battle fought on a knife's edge.

How can I blame them, when I know that what was done to me was also done to them? When I know that part of being tortured and brainwashed in cults involves implicating the abused child and the abused adolescent in the torture, brainwashing and killing of others?

Acceptance of the reality of ritual abuse allows for no neat divisions between victim and perpetrator. No one can be squeaky clean any more. Denial and emotional abandonment are just as destructive to life, sanity and liberty as are open hostility and violence.

To accept the reality of ritual abuse questions the foundations of our ethics and morality. It highlights the woeful inadequacies of our 'justice' system. Above all, acceptance of the reality of ritual abuse means accepting that the world is a far more dangerous place than we had previously thought. Far worse things happen daily—and especially nightly—to adults, adolescents, children and babies than we have ever allowed ourselves to imagine.

Miriam Wainwright

◆

The most horrific, unbelievably terrifying, brutal memories hit me when I was 48 years old: I had had three little babies born to me who were killed in rituals.

Babies are a sign of hope. But hope was never mine. My mind closed the door on all this. I shut down all my emotions.

The effects of the ritual abuse on my personality were terrible. I had to be perfect. I had a perfect house, a perfect husband and perfect children. I was overprotective with my children. I had to get out of bed every night to see they were safe even when they were teenagers. I couldn't make friends. I didn't need anything. I just existed.

So how does one become a warm, caring, human person again? For me it has been a lot of hard work, a lot of determination to heal and to reclaim what was robbed from me.

The hardest thing was that very few people wanted to hear about my memories, and even fewer could believe them. To me that is the most important thing—that we can talk about our truths and be validated, no matter how terrible our story.

I know I am responsible for my own healing. That was a hard lesson to learn, but once I had learned it my life became somewhat easier. I began listening to my inner selves, and they have started to respond. Support has come.

Today I can make and keep friends. I know they love me. We ritual abuse survivors are healing and speaking out.

Sally Bateman

◆

The irony for me as a ritual abuse survivor is that the past never seems to stay behind. Even though I tried very hard to suppress them, the memories of ritual abuse in childhood came flooding in. I have always been aware of having been ritually abused in adolescence and early adulthood.

Our parents were respected, socially active members of the community, and we attended private school. The masks we all wore were readily accepted by society, just as those same masks, so painfully worn today by myself and other ritual abuse survivors, are also rarely questioned.

The refusal to gaze on the darkest side of humanity retraumatises and isolates us in our pain. We have so few places to turn, so few safe houses in which to hide, so few brave souls prepared to support us through our torment. Too often we are tossed in the 'too hard' basket. This adds to our guilt and shame. And we are forced to place economic survival before our emotional healing. For those of us still trapped in the spider web of cult, not only are we ostracised by an outraged society, we are often shunned by fellow survivors. But heal we do!

Jain Robbins

✦

I am a 39-year-old woman. I experienced 18 years of prolonged and repeated torture and betrayal. I was horrifically abused by my mother, my father, grandparents, aunts, uncles, older cousins, and other respected members of our community.

People who had the responsibility of nurturing and protecting me, betrayed me. They tortured me in every conceivable way. I was coerced into making impossible life and death choices. I was never safe. I was not allowed to own anything, not even a toy. They said I was nothing. They said I would never escape. They said I belonged to them. They said they would find me and kill me. They said I was useless and mad. They said I was a liar and murderer. They said I would rot from the inside out. They impregnated me and murdered my children.

And I have survived.

Two people close to me believed my truth and supported me through my devastation, my pain, my deep shame, my guilt, my loss, my rage. I have learned new, positive ways of seeing myself, my power, my reality and my value.

And I reckon that is not too bad.

The outrage of ritual abuse can survive only as long as people turn a blind eye to it. Being believed and loved was an important part of my healing process, along with my own courage and determination. Cults are not inherently powerful. They are powerful only when they have absolute control over their victims, and when they have our compliance in refusing to acknowledge and act upon their existence.

Grace McInnerny

✦

The photographs on this and the following pages are of some of the contributors to this book, taken at the age when they were first abused.

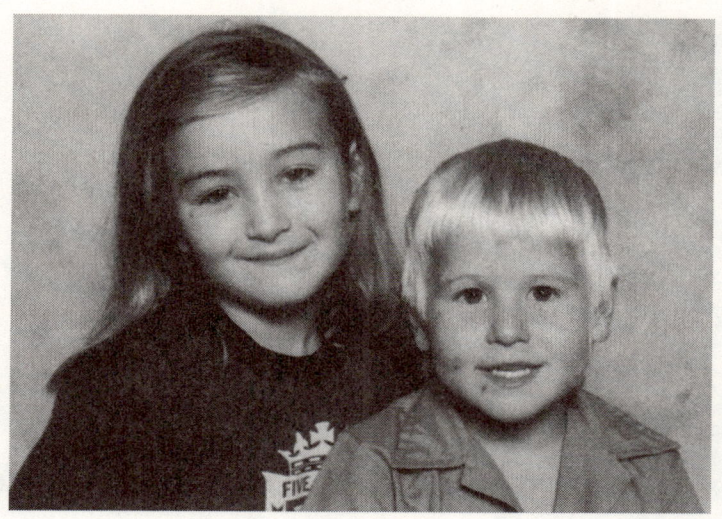

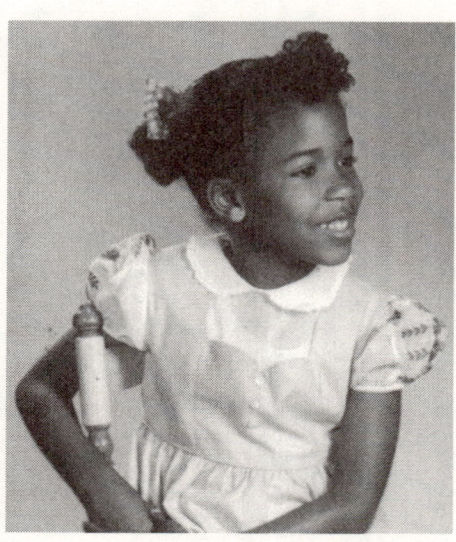

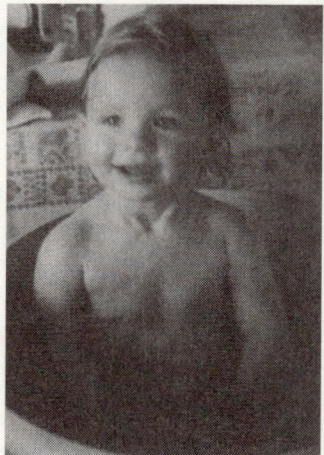

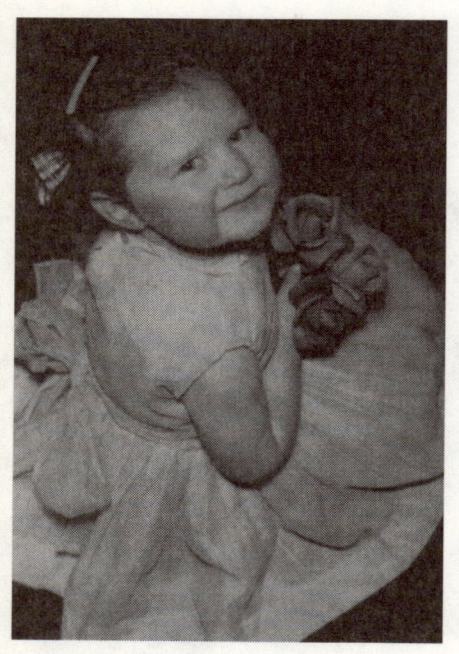

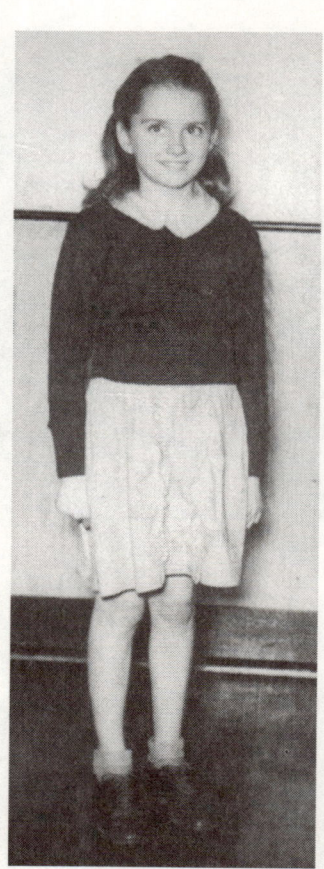

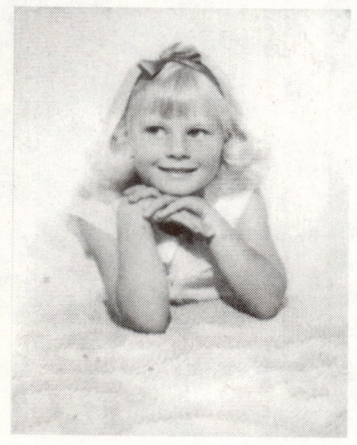

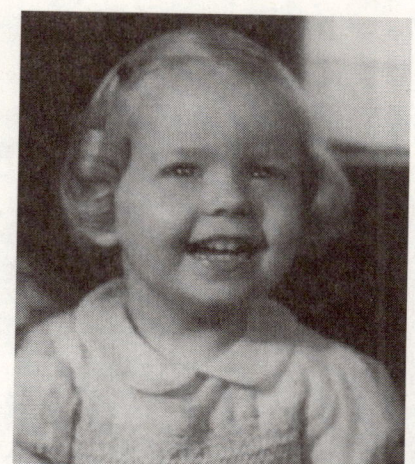

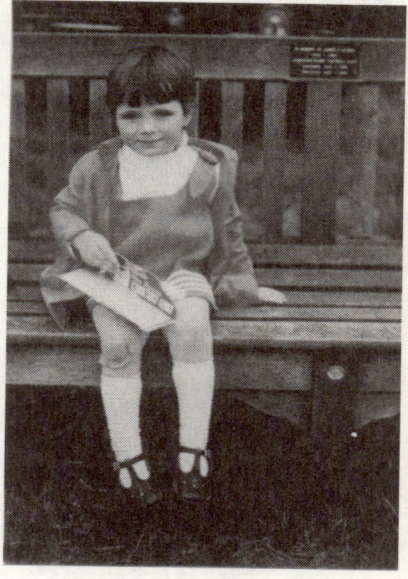

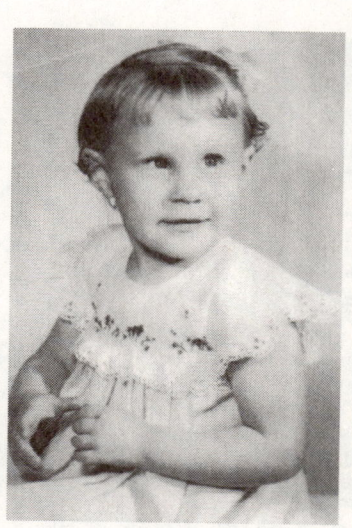

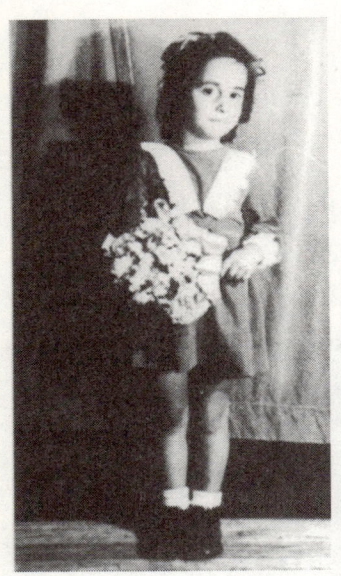

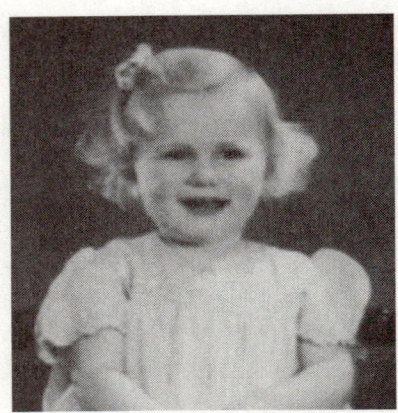

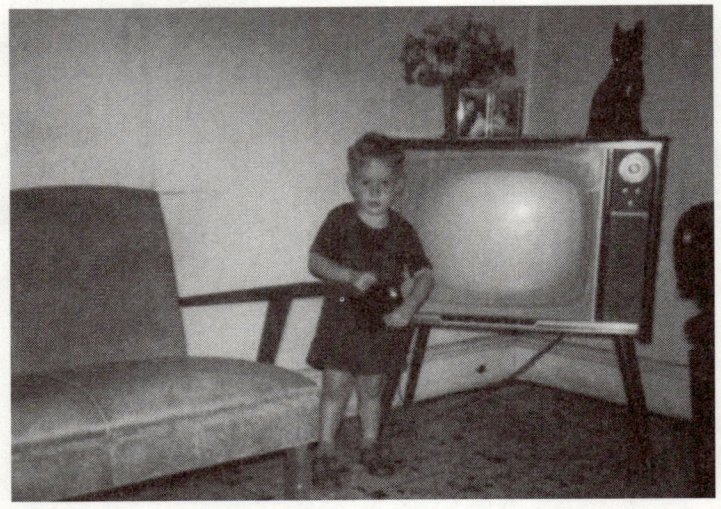

CHAPTER FIVE

✦

Breaking the silence

If you bring forth what is within you, what you bring forth will save you. If you do not bring forth what is within you, what you do not bring forth will destroy you.

Gospel of Thomas

It takes so much courage to break the silence. Telling someone the truth about what happened to you means accepting the truth that you were abused. At ASCA we liken it to an alcoholic joining AA. It is the beginning of your healing. Until you tell someone, the pain sits inside you, it can destroy you. Released, you are freed, you become a survivor not a victim, and you begin to live.

But it is hard to admit, even to yourself, the truth about your childhood if you have been indoctrinated with lies that lead to deep, abiding feelings of guilt, shame and fear. Threats made to children are intended to frighten them into keeping the truth a secret. These are usually so effective that most of us never told anyone what was happening to us. As adults the fear we felt when we were young still exercises its power, as it was intended to do.

However frightened you may still feel, it is important to remember that you are no longer a child, no longer helpless and dependent. We adult survivors can challenge the old lies, we can seek help. By breaking the injunction of silence, we can break the power of our abusers and so help others as well as ourselves.

As long as you feel you must remain silent, to some extent the abuser still maintains power, still 'owns' you. And for all the current concern about child abuse, people cannot believe that this has happened throughout history: that for every child now being helped, there is an adult who has been suffering in silence since childhood. For every child now being helped, there will be another child who cannot tell, as we could not tell. Each of us can help to challenge the idea that child abuse is a recent issue, or that it is easy to tell.

It is important that all of us who are able to break the silence should do so, and not only for our own sake. While we remain silent, those for whom it is not safe to tell will feel more isolated and alone. While we remain silent, those who love us will not be able to understand and help us. While we remain silent, the public will not learn. While we remain silent, the next generation will not benefit from the way we have faced our pain. While we remain silent, child abuse will go on and on.

TELLING OUR TRUTH

Breaking the silence may be the most important step of all in the journey towards healing, and it is not something to undertake lightly. Who to tell and when to tell is a decision each of us has to make for ourselves. But don't underestimate the importance of ensuring that, when the time to tell comes, you feel safe, you are supported, and you are well prepared. Choose someone you trust.

Before telling your family you may find it safer to tell ASCA, a caring survivor friend, or, most likely of all, your therapist—someone who understands about child abuse and is more likely to respond positively. Once you have broken the silence, you are on the path to healing and you will gain the strength to tell others, including your family.

Telling the family is never easy. As survivors we need more love and support from our family than other people, so a lack of understanding from them, their rejection or denial of our truth, can be devastating. In families where there are generations of abuse, secrecy is likely to be very strong and any challenge to it seen as deeply threatening. In non-abusive families, there may still be a lack of understanding, warmth and empathy, and difficulties dealing with painful truths. People do not want to believe that someone they love can have been hurt, or that they failed as parents to protect, so the easiest course of action is to deny the truth of what you are telling them. Accept this possibility before you speak to your family, then tell if you want to.

The agonising question 'Should I tell my children about my past?' is one that all survivors who are parents will sooner or later ask themselves. Part of breaking the silence is to break the shame and the secrets that are carried down the generations. It is particularly important to tell your children if they are in contact with the person who abused you. Many ASCA members have to deal with the pain of realising that their children have been abused by the same person who abused them. As survivors, we try to minimise and forget what happened to us. But we must not do this when it comes to giving access to offenders. They are unlikely to have changed; offenders cannot be trusted. Even if you can't tell your children the full story, protect them by telling them as much as they are capable of understanding. Children can learn from our pain.

My heart was pounding, my hands were shaking, I was spacing out, my headache was so bad I thought I would explode as I reached for the phone. I had dialled the number so many times in the last week, but then lost the courage to speak. Why was it so hard?

A woman answered. I managed to say that I had been abused as a child by a teacher when I was eight. The woman told me I was so brave to phone. I felt such relief: she understood, she knew how difficult it had been for me. From the depths of me I started to cry. The pain was being let out.

I will always be grateful to that first person I told, at the end of the ASCA phone line. I slept that night better than I've slept in years, and the next day the headache eased. I'm on the journey now and it can't be worse than where I was before.

Jill Harting

◆

When I first began to recover my memories I was so shocked and bewildered I couldn't understand what was happening, and was unable either to believe or not to believe what my mind and my body were telling me. I wrote down the fragments of memory as they returned until I could finally piece it all together. I'd been having therapy for more than a year, but the idea of telling my therapist what I'd finally found out simply terrified me. I couldn't do it. I didn't ask myself why not, I was just aware that whenever I pictured myself talking to him about it, I was filled with this overwhelming fear. In the end I took my journal with me, and gave it to him to read. We sat in silence for almost the whole session, while he read my story.

I knew that I hadn't discovered everything I needed to know. Over the next few weeks, more memories returned. Finally, I remembered the injunction I'd been given that I should never ever tell anyone, and the threat that I'd be killed if I did. Once I'd remembered that—and remembering was itself terrifying—I realised why I hadn't been able to tell. And I also realised that only by daring to tell now would I break the power of the injunction that I'd been living under for more than 40 years. I went to the next session so afraid I was trembling all over. I whispered what had happened—and waited for the thunderbolt to strike. He said, very gently, 'You've told me, and you're still alive. The fear they created they could use in the threat against a child, but not an adult. It is no longer possible for them to harm you. Your adult self can protect your child self now. They can't hurt you.'

I felt completely exhausted after the session, but later that day as I went for a walk in the spring sunshine I felt a sense of release and was filled with a joy I'd never known before. There were many struggles still ahead, but that was the turning point for me.

Candida Hunt

◆

SILENCE IS NOT GOLDEN
Silence!
Silence is golden
and deadly.
It speaks
thunderously,
ominously
of that which is to come.

When peace
is shattered
and hope
evaporates.

When fear
envelops
the heart
struggling
to be free.

Silence
is golden
for you

Not me.

Silence!

Gillian Graham

✦

The first time I talked to a friend about incest I said too much at
once, and I think she was pretty shocked and overwhelmed. She

didn't really understand, and didn't want to be involved in my healing. It took a long time for me to understand that she wasn't rejecting me as a person. We are still friends, but aren't as close as we once were and we don't discuss issues relating to abuse. Saying a lot initially to her was inconsiderate on my part.

Lynette Adams

◆

From a man's point of view telling is even harder because the fear of disclosure connects to the fear of society categorising you as being gay, and that you asked for it, because they see it as a sexual thing and not as an abuse of power. It can be scary, yet the love and caring that has come back to me has made it worth the struggle.

Now I can look back and say I'm glad I spoke out and broke the secrecy, and the power of that secrecy over me, for where I am in my life now is influenced by connecting in a loving way with others—those who want to listen, understand, share and grow in knowledge as we work to free ourselves from oppressive abusive practices.

Paul Philips

◆

I have a problem with anger. It frightens me greatly because it reminds me of my mother—enraged, out of control, abusive. I cannot tolerate it in myself for fear of being like her. During the course of my counselling, my therapist taught me some safe anger release techniques—beating pillows and so on. It was a harrowing experience for me, to admit that I had feelings of anger and to let those feelings out. As a child, I adopted silence as a survival strategy.

When I finally managed to beat up the pillows with some conviction, my therapist said, 'Well, that was really good, but how about trying it again, and this time make a noise.' I was shocked.

In my mind I had been screaming, loudly. But it was only in my mind. I didn't realise that I had not uttered a sound as I vented my rage. I couldn't believe it. Still silent after all these years—my voice taken away from me by the horror of my childhood.

Around the same time, I started doing some a capella singing workshops, just for fun. Within a year I had joined a gospel and spiritual singing group which performed regularly, and the opportunity for the group to do a tour of churches and schools in Vanuatu came up. A film crew came with us to make a documentary of the tour—including individual interviews of all the singers. This was a scary prospect to an ordinary girl like me, especially one who had been a shy, terrified child.

But as you may have found in your own journey, things happen for a reason. Throughout the trip I had a feeling of being exactly where I was supposed to be and doing exactly what was right for me at the time. So I was determined to be totally honest about my answers in the interview when asked how I got involved in singing, how it made me feel, why I did it.

I talked about what singing means to me. How I found my voice again. Not just to sing, but to speak out. And especially to speak out about abuse and its devastating effect on so many lives. I spoke about how glad I was that I had somehow hung in there and that the creative side of me was not broken or dead, as I had thought. As a child, I had been denied opportunities to perform in school plays or choirs. But that spark was still alive within me, demanding an outlet, crying out for expression, and the child inside me was desperate to be heard—in joy as well as in pain. I spoke about how singing for me is an affirmation. It is a statement of my aliveness and spirit—the fact that I am still here. I have survived.

I wanted to take the opportunity so strangely presented to me by that interview to encourage other survivors of abuse not to give up hope, not to give up their dreams. I wanted to encourage them to feel triumphant about having survived at all, to search for the goodness inside themselves no matter what they had to do to survive and no matter what had been done to them. I wanted to encourage my fellow survivors to find their voice again.

Joan Burns

◆

When I remembered, the first thing I did was tell. At first it was easy for me to tell family and friends because to begin with I didn't have any distress about the memory. Several weeks after disclosing I had a delayed reaction of absolute terror and hysteria, which made any further attempts at disclosure far more difficult.

I've never regretted telling workmates, friends and casual acquaintances. I seemed to understand that the more I spoke about it the more real it became and the easier it was to deal with. Abuse is usually a very secretive issue, and discussing it eased the pain of it. The majority of people were sympathetic. I feel it has been an advantage to discuss openly the fact that I'm in counselling for child abuse, as it is one less secret to bear.

Through healing I've discovered that secrets are devastating and can kill you (that is, lead to suicide), and the more often you say it out loud the less of a secret it is. If we keep it secret, how will society ever learn the truth?

Lyn

◆

I was three years old when I was sexually abused by a cousin at Christmas.

The first person I told—in 1980, when I was 20 years old—was my girlfriend. She confronted me and asked me if I had been sexually abused, and I said yes, as a matter of fact I had been. She was very supportive, comforting and understanding, but I was numb about it. I'd left the skeleton in the closet for so long, and the abuse was so ingrained in my psyche.

It took me another eight years before I could tell my mum, and her reaction was great. There was no hesitation or doubt in her mind that I was telling the truth, because she knew me well enough to know I wouldn't lie about something like that. This was my turning point. It lifted a monumental weight off my mind because the abuser was a member of my mother's family, and I was so relieved after talking to her.

I felt so ashamed for a long time, but now I don't care who knows as I feel I've got nothing to hide. If more people speak out—especially males—then we know we are not alone, and there's no shame because there's nothing to be ashamed about. Would you feel ashamed if you were in a car accident? Incest, paedophilia, mental illness—these are the last taboos in Western society. Of all my friends, I had a bad reaction from only one, and as a result of my disclosure some of my male friends opened up and told me they'd been through the same thing.

Real men show emotion because it's part of the human condition. Real men do cry if the need arises, because it releases a little bit of the pressure. Keeping it inside makes you more of a victim— speaking out lets people know that it's more common than people think. By speaking out we won't stop the perpetrators, but we will make them think twice.

By speaking out and learning more about what happened to me I am learning to understand myself and the reactions to things from the past. My sexual orientation is heterosexual, and admitting what happened to me was a big step because some people would have branded me homosexual; maybe they're not sure of their own sexuality. I feel that it's a stumbling block for men coming forward about the crime that was committed against them.

David Cox

◆

I have always had a feeling of aloneness. As an illegitimate wartime baby, I was removed from my mother at birth and placed in a series of institutions until I was adopted at seven. These places were not pleasant, and nor were the people running them. They knew that illegitimate children had no one to defend them and they exploited this. But I was sure that I had put that part of my life behind me. I now have a wonderful family—30 years of marriage and two beautiful daughters, one of whom has recently moved into working in the area of child abuse. That was how I came to be watching Liz Mullinar on *The Midday Show* last year.

Hearing Liz talk about her abuse and how it affected her really touched a chord in me. I too suffered from irrational fears—the dark, going to sleep. When my daughter Jacqui came home I really wanted to talk about myself; for the first time, I thought that I could relate to being a 'survivor'. Talking about my childhood was rather frightening but also quite a relief. I had *never* talked about it before. My husband and children learned not to ask me any questions because they would get shrugged off. But seeing Liz released something in me.

It felt bizarre to open up the blocks I had set in place. For nearly 50 years I had remained silent, so I felt at first as if I was talking about someone else. I felt removed from myself because I was scared. Scared to admit that I may have issues resulting from my childhood that I had chosen not to deal with.

I'm glad I watched the show that day and learned that someone else understood me and how I felt. Talking to my daughter was rewarding. She made me realise that perhaps I do have unresolved issues. Talking about them is a sort of a relief, and I feel I am doing some good in letting others know how the other half have lived.

Rosemary Manning

◆

'Never tell' was the message I received loud and clear throughout my abuse, though it was never put into words. It was never an option. When my father acted as though everything was 'normal' in our 'happy family', how could I even begin to put into words the terror of my hidden life? The life that was filled with such shame and confusion existed alongside my ordinary, everyday life. I went to the beach and to Brownies and to school and to friends' parties, without ever thinking of telling anyone what happened to me sometimes when my father and I were alone.

When I recovered the memories of my childhood abuse, I carried this shame and confusion into my present life. I found it humiliating to tell my therapist about even the most 'minor' incident of abuse. I didn't tell my friends, and I couldn't tell my family.

Joining an incest survivors group helped me to voice my experiences. For the first time I was able to find validation of the significance of what had happened to me, from others who had experienced similar things. I had never even labelled the abuse 'incest' until I joined this group, and the others there helped me see that incest takes many forms, and does not just apply to vaginal rape. I began to see that I was justified in being hurt by what had happened, and more than that, that it was OK to tell people. There was no further threat to me, the adult.

Mono

◆

Silence is not golden, it is oppressive, and can cause more harm than good when you're reuniting yourself to your lost feelings and emotions. To those who don't understand how unhealthy it is to stifle your emotions, I'd say, don't stifle us any further by saying, 'What's past is done, there's no point in talking about it now'. That attitude is damaging to people who already have a low estimate of themselves.

We all have a right to our own beliefs, our own self-expression. To me, silence means not being able to express myself. To express myself, I need to be in touch with the reality of my past. I do not need people telling me that my past is unimportant or trivial. It is all part of my make-up, part of who I am.

Diana Beth

◆

As I was sitting on my bedroom floor I was overwhelmed with my life's nightmares. I did not want to believe that my grandfather had raped me several times when I was a child. But I had to believe it. I was being tormented by nightmares and overwhelming feelings. I was so scared and alone. I knew that if was to survive I had to tell someone.

With hindsight I now realise that I had been suffering the more noticeable effects of the abuse since high school. It was having a terrible impact on my relationships, and I was becoming more and more withdrawn, depressed and suicidal. I was really in a desperate situation; I was choosing between life and death.

A man I had met at uni told me he wanted to get to know me because he liked my style. His name was Andrew, and I knew he would be worth knowing. The only problem was that I could not trust him. I could not trust him with my feelings or my body. Whenever we were alone I imagined him hurting me. He never tried to touch me without asking, and in my mind I knew that he would never hurt me, but I was still petrified of him. I knew it was because of the abuse, and I knew that if I didn't do something I would lose him and my last hope of survival.

I was so alone. I would lie awake each night crying, hurting so deeply. My heart ached for the loss of my innocence, for the little girl who had not been protected. She was so alone and scared. I had to break the cycle of silence. Break out from the fear and tell someone. Then I would be the one in control, not my abuser.

My silence towards Andrew was pushing him farther and farther away. I desperately wanted him to understand me. I wrote him a letter telling him my fears, my feelings and a little of the events of the abuse. I sat there while he read the letter. My heart pounded as I thought of him rejecting me or my claims. I was so scared. After his eyes left the paper, they were filled with tears and pain. He asked if he could hold me. We cried as we held each other. For the first time in my life I felt completely safe.

Since that day he has been there to drive me to counselling, support me, listen to me, believe me, love me and hold me. Since that day I have not been alone. He helped me through my last two years of uni, and I now have a job as a registered nurse. He has helped me to stay alive, taught me that I am of worth, that I'm strong, smart and beautiful.

I realise how very lucky I am. I have told other people too, family and friends. Most of them reacted in a very destructive way, but I felt I had to tell them. They were my friends and I had to break the silence, stop keeping secrets. Telling people about the abuse was one of the hardest things I've had to do, but it was worth telling all those people in order to find one who gave me what I needed.

Kate

◆

After the death of my father in a plane crash, my mother married a violent, abusive, bullying lawyer. I well know the sheer terror of just coming home from school, of literally living in fear ... Of sitting in the back yard, frozen, in the middle of winter until bedtime to avoid the closed fist smashed into the face.

Looking at [abused children], I remembered the helplessness and the humiliation of being kicked and punched, of having nowhere to turn, of being at the mercy of a monster. Most of all, I remembered the shame. No one ever spoke of what was happening and, in a small town in New Zealand, everyone knew. I did not speak of it to my three brothers or sister for another 10 years. I still weep sometimes for that bruised and needy little girl that I was ... always in trouble at school, crying out for help.

Violence devastated my family. Shared among my brothers and sister—all very bright—is violent behaviour, alcoholism, drug abuse, unfulfilled potential, difficulty in sustaining relationships.

My brother Hugh committed suicide years ago, at the age of 26. His last words to a friend were, 'I feel worthless.' Ours was a shared history and his death broke my heart. If only someone in charge had shown compassion to a little boy who cried 'Help me, help me, help me' every night in his sleep.

Susan Chenery

◆

Speaking out has been one of the most profoundly healing and terrifying things I have done in my life. I choose to be part of the solution, and do not want to be part of any hidden conspiracy of secrecy and silence which only enables child sexual abuse to flourish. I broke the golden rule that incest families create, which is not to talk about our family business.

Through my own experience I have come to understand that incest families are a complicated web. Trying to get out of the stranglehold of enmeshment and power my parents had was like trying to find my way through a maze. It was hard leaving a dysfunctional family, as I had to grow out of my childhood fantasy of trying to get my parents' love and feeling responsible for everything. I'm happy to say that I am much healthier now and am becoming emotionally mature.

When my memories came up, a well-meaning friend suggested that I speak to my mother as she might be able to help me. This friend had no understanding of the dynamics of sexual abuse in families, and at the time nor did I. When I spoke to my mother she completely denied everything, even the daily episodes that went on in my home. It was then that I realised my mother had known all along, and had been covering everything up. To make matters worse, although I told her not to tell my father as I wanted to face him myself, and not to tell my sister as I was concerned because she was pregnant at the time, she betrayed me once again to try and save herself; she became very controlling and manipulative.

The fact that she did this devastated me. I discovered that my mother would do anything to prevent the truth being brought out in the open. She scapegoated me, and tried every trick in the book, even implying that it was the vitamins I was taking, or people planting ideas in my head. When I did a personal development course to heal my wounded self-esteem, she used the false memory myth against me, said I had chronic fatigue syndrome (which I have never had), implied I was crazy, etc. It is easy to see why so many people end up in mental institutions because of child abuse.

I was blessed to be validated by a schoolteacher who had taught me when I was 11 years old. At a chance meeting just after I recovered my memories of being sexually abused, she confirmed that she had been very worried about me as my handwriting had gone really weird at that time, and she could not understand it. I don't remember that year at school at all; I blocked it out completely.

I have found it very enlightening telling friends. One of my best friends, who I thought would support me and who knew my family, was shocked, disbelieved me and became quite angry. She told me to forget about it, which was the worst thing she could have said because that's what I had done all my life and it wasn't working for me any longer. However, another friend who I hadn't thought would be supportive showed so much love and compassion, believing me and helping me talk about it.

My sister was in denial when I told her, and didn't want to face it, but after two years came back and told me that I was right and that something had happened to her too. She is now getting counselling as well.

I am a much stronger person now for daring to speak the truth around this taboo subject. I have come to realise that my parents are very wounded people, but pretending nothing happened hadn't solved anything—it had only created sickness and worse problems. It has been important for me to speak out.

From my own experience I recommend that you speak to a counsellor first before you tell anyone else, because there is no way of knowing how people will react. Be prepared for the unexpected, and think carefully about what it is you want to say. I believe it is best to say a little at first and see how the person reacts. I don't believe there is any right or wrong time to do so, though you do need to feel that you can cope with the negative response if it doesn't go well.

Do it in your own time when you feel ready. It is advisable to have support afterwards as it could bring up a lot of emotional responses. Seeking professional advice is very helpful. Stand strong in your truth, and don't let anyone persuade you about how you should feel or get you to back down because they don't want to face the ugliness of it all. Create a healthy support network around you of people who will validate you and not deny it or brush it aside. You may even find that other people who have been abused find the courage to come forward too.

Lies and secrecy make the mind, body and soul sick, and create an unhealthy environment to live in. I am healthier since I have spoken out. Before, I was always getting sick because I was suppressing everything. Light and truth will always win over darkness in the long run. When each one of us talks about it, we light a torch for truth to lead a way through the darkness to a better world, and save our children from abuse.

Linda Honey

✦

Telling my family was the hardest part. When I first decided to confront my father about one memory of abuse, I felt I should tell my mother and brother first, and did so. They were very supportive, and despite their shock they affirmed their belief in me and my memory and promised to stand by me. As time went on and I found the strength to confront my father about more memories, usually in the context of family meetings, my mother and brother continued to support and believe me, despite my father's blanket denial.

My mother supports me in many ways, and I especially appreciate the fact that I can talk with her about my memories of abuse. She stands by me and does not believe my father's denial. Yet I find it difficult that she remains married to him. At the same time though, I can see that to leave him after 30 years of marriage would be a huge step, and it's a step I would like her to make for her own reasons, not for mine, if at all.

Most of all, I appreciate her encouragement to 'tell'. When I wrote my life story in a collection of accounts of incest survivors, she said she read it, went for a walk and cried for me. It has been difficult for her, yet she still supports me in my need to tell my story. She wasn't able to be there for me as a child in the way I would have liked, for whatever reason. Yet now that I have trusted her with my pain, she has come through for me. And I know that she gives me more strength to keep on going, because she encourages me to speak. And it is only through speaking and speaking and speaking that I will break through the threat, 'Never tell!'

Mono

◆

I always remembered being sexually abused by my grandfather at about the age of six. When I was 11, my parents, brothers, sister and I were at the dinner table. Dad was pissed as usual, and was into a monologue about how great his dad was. With no planning, I said, 'No he's not—he used to molest me!' Dad was shocked and angry—at me. He said, 'How dare you talk like that at the dinner table? Go to your room!'

The next thing I recall, I am lying on my bed in the dark and feeling absolutely nothing. One big nothing. Mum comes in and sits by me. She asks gently, 'Did he hurt you—did you bleed?' I reply in the negative, and she pats me on the arm. 'Oh, you'll be right,' she says, and walks away.

The whole thing got buried in me, though not forgotten. I couldn't say anything about it, not until I was 23 and going for help about my drinking.

At 25 and sober, I am relating the dinner table scene to a counsellor. Suddenly I am overcome by the deepest grief. I don't cry—I howl loudly. I howl and howl and can't stop. I cry my heart out.

Being sober, it wasn't hard to connect to my feelings, the ones I don't remember feeling as a child. There was so much grief in me.

I told my father about Grandpa again when I was about 25. His reaction was different this time—he believed me, and was upset for my sake.

Wendy Nelson

◆

My sexual abuse began when I was three years old, and I eventually told my mother. She said, 'I don't want to hear about it.' So I learned that what happened to me didn't matter very much. However, it began to play on my mind somewhat when I was having my first child at 15.

I asked my mother if she remembered. She said to me that I'd always been a flirtatious child, climbing all over men, and that they couldn't be blamed. Many years later, when I started my healing process, I told her about other assaults I'd experienced. She screamed at me not to tell her. I think my mistake lay in assuming that now we were both adults she'd listen to me.

I would suggest to any survivor contemplating disclosure that they consider the cost, and be open to the possibility of not getting what they might be looking for. I believe cruel, blaming or insensitive responses create a secondary wound, and sometimes I feel glad that there are certain things I did not tell my mother, as I don't have more secondary wounds.

The trouble is that it was extremely difficult for a time to tell anyone, as I was sure that everyone would respond in the same way as my mother—her cold, angry eyes full of disgust for me. In terms of nurturing and support, I have come to believe that it is the substance, not the source that counts. When a friend drops in a little gift, when my therapist hears me, or when someone hugs me, these are all 'mother-like' acts. I have selected my own 'family', as it were, people I can tell anything to, and I know that with these people I am not opening my precious self to re-wounding.

The child inside me also learns that there are different ways that people respond. This is tremendously healing. I can look into the eyes of these people as I tell them. Sometimes I still see anger and disgust, but it's not for me, it's for those who hurt me.

Louise Plummer

◆

When I told my parents my mother was absorbed with self-pity. 'I can't believe this is happening to me,' she said. My father was going to approach the perpetrators and 'get an apology'. Within a week of my telling them they had asked the neighbours whether it happened, asked the local doctor if he believed it could have happened, and seen a social worker who advised them to get more 'accurate' details, because it was probably exaggerated.

They quickly went into denial. My mother was devastated by my accusations. They approached the perpetrators, meeting with denial from them. In the six and a half years since I told my parents they have decided I've been brainwashed by the church, and they don't understand why I am 'doing this to the family'.

About ten months ago I received, out of the blue, a solicitor's letter advising me of a defamation case brought by one of my brothers—one of the abusers. I was told to retract the statements I had made to my parents accusing my brother, or court action would follow. I refused to do this. Over the next few weeks we anxiously awaited advice from my solicitor, who had never heard of a defamation case within a family before.

I agreed not to discuss the abuse with anyone except legal advisors and my counsellor for the interim. I eventually said that I would not retract my statement, and I would continue to talk to whom I wished, and I heard nothing more from his solicitor—no reply at all. My husband's family were as supportive as they could be. I think my telling them was like 'joining the dots' for them.

Juley Taben

◆

The end of 1994 was probably the biggest step I took in disclosure. I sent a letter to all my relatives about what had taken place in the family house where I grew up. Why? Because I was sick and tired of the labelling and innuendoes I was being subjected to by some of them. I have been attacked because of my single status, my quietness and shyness, etc. But above all, I was tired of the truth being kept a secret. I believe that secrets such as abuse should not be swept under the carpet.

I told them in the letter what took place, and how it had affected me. That that is why I am the way I am—it is not from choice. I also told them about my suicidal intentions, a consequence of my experiences in childhood. By speaking out to the relatives I felt slightly freer in myself, in that I broke the veil of secrecy. Enough was enough!

I subsequently received no support or encouragement. But the fact remains that I did it. The letter took courage and strength, and I have no regrets. Little Janice was finally being given a voice— that quiet little girl had never had one before.

It's time to break the code of silence, to be the voice for all to be heard and break the cycle of abuse. As the song by Susan Aglukark says, no one has to 'Suffer in Silence'. Writing this is another way of Little Janice being heard—thank you for listening.

Janice Atkinson

◆

My mother had never shown me any love or affection. I tried to tell her about my father, but she would never listen—she'd just say she hated me and tell me to go away. I had the courage to confront her only a year ago, to ask her if she really knew what my father had done. After much ranting and raving she retaliated by saying yes, she knew, and I deserved what I got. This to me was as traumatic as the abuse. I still can't believe that she did nothing to help or protect me.

Jenny Lacey

◆

I am a police officer in my late twenties. When I was a boy I was abused by a cousin who had endeared himself so much to my immediate family that he almost belonged in it. The abuse stopped when I was in my early teens, and then I got on with my life— not forgetting about the abuse, but certainly not addressing it.

A couple of years ago I started to question why I had been unable to commit to relationships and always found myself alone. I then started to allow memories of my past to surface, and found that I was unable to think of much else. During a visit from an aunt I learnt of abuse that had taken place within her generation, and I found myself telling her about my own abuse.

I didn't tell her any specific details, but I found great relief in someone else actually knowing what had happened to me. A short time later I told my flatmate—a close friend—and remember that while I was telling her I was sitting on the couch, crying uncontrollably, and not allowing her to hug me or show me any affection.

I sought professional help, but unfortunately I didn't trust him so I decided to go it alone. I found myself being completely consumed and obsessed by my abuse. I was telling all my friends and anyone who would reassure me that it wasn't my fault. I was becoming depressed more often, and found solace in alcohol. Outwardly, of course, I didn't allow anyone to know I wasn't coping; as always, outwardly I appeared to be strong and in control.

Then one night I found myself on the couch with my service revolver in my hand. I was debating whether it was worth continuing, and I still don't know what convinced me not to put an end to it all. But I decided there and then that I needed help. I sought the help of the police psychologist. After a couple of sessions I had a burning need to go home to tell my mum and dad of the abuse, and to receive a hug from them. I needed to hear my parents tell me they loved me, that they believed me, that it wasn't my fault.

Since telling my parents I know they love me very much. They believe me without doubt, and certainly reassure me that my cousin is the person at fault. My parents feel some guilt about having allowed him access to me as a child. I know my news has hurt them a lot, but I also know it has answered many questions about me that they had over the years. I know they are glad I've told them, and we all now enjoy the honesty we share.

My flatmate, my aunt, my brothers and sister and my closest friends have all stood by me through truly horrible times. I often question why they continue to support me—they must see things in me that I can't see. I'm so grateful to them for being there for me, not offering advice or trying to understand, but just being there. Without their support I would never have made it this far, or found the strength I've needed to pull through. On a bad day I remind myself that what I'm going through is nothing compared to the times I'd suffered alone, and that the worst day of my life was the first day of my recovery.

Tony

◆

Learning to deal with the truth and pain of my childhood was almost as difficult as living it. How I must have appeared to my children is anyone's guess. I know my mood swings were extreme, I was over-protective, and giving my children all the love I was denied was paramount. I was often depressed, and the house reflected my inner turmoil and lack of self-esteem.

Keeping the children abreast of all our family situations was better than the secrets of my childhood. Besides, children are very good at seeing past the facade we adults erect around ourselves, pretending to ourselves that 'nobody knows what's going on'.

Once I began therapy, the need to speak about my childhood, the truth about my life, became increasingly important to my healing process. I had stopped contact with my father and sister, the only family left, and the need to explain to my girls why there were so many changes became most important. My daughters were about 11 and eight years old when I told them, as easily as I could,

'When I was a little girl my daddy touched me where he shouldn't'. I went on to explain that it had made me feel bad about myself, and how much my father had hurt me. I told them I was talking to someone who could help me, and that we wouldn't be seeing my family again. I also let them know that if they didn't understand everything I'd said, it was okay to ask me questions about it any time they wanted.

I feel it is important to tell our children for many reasons. As survivors, we know how destructive secrets and silence can be, so why continue such a painful cycle with our children? Being open and honest with them teaches them that sharing feelings and difficult life situations is a healthy way to resolve problems. By sharing with our children our deepest pain, we are showing them the respect we did not receive as children, we are teaching them about trust.

Revealing my 'secret' helped them to understand why I was so passionate about their right to privacy, why I was so careful to teach them that their own bodies were special, and how to keep themselves safe and protected. I still believe knowledge is protection, and that what happened to me is less likely to happen to them as a result. Incest is cruel, vicious and has long-lasting effects. I'll carry its scars forever. It needs to be discussed openly, for in an open, honest atmosphere secrets can't be harboured, nor will abuse be tolerated.

Janina Malone

◆

Often the hardest decision is when and what to tell the children, as our natural wish is to shield them from the pain and the hurt. I didn't have to make that difficult decision—it was impossible to keep my pain from the children. They now tell me they really didn't understand exactly what was going on at the time, but the knowledge of what happened to me has been a great learning experience for them in their own relationships.

My younger son, who is 17, gave a talk at his school to his Year 12 mates, and told them about the effects of sexual abuse on his mother. I was so proud: proud because he feels no shame—nor should he—and proud because it means that if we tell our children, we dispel the shame for the next generation. His friends will accept and know that sexual abuse can happen to anyone, and there is no shame in having endured it. When my other son's girlfriend was having difficulties relating to him sexually, he was able to understand, and to ask her if she had suffered from sexual abuse. She felt enormous relief that here was a boy who understood her problem and did not condemn her for it.

Liz Mullinar

✦

I knew that there were skeletons in my family's cupboard, though it took me a long time to come to terms with the fact that I was one of them. A wise friend said that one of the ways in which I could stop the shadow of abuse falling on future generations would be to bring the skeleton out of the cupboard: to tell my children. They had grown up having to cope with my mood swings and long periods of depression, and although I did my best to appear 'normal' with them, I knew that with children's sensitivity and instinctive empathy they were troubled, and would have sensed that something was wrong. They knew that I didn't get on with one of my sisters and my older brother, and that I found both my parents very difficult; they knew my childhood had been emotionally damaging.

In the end, the decision about when to tell them of the sexual abuse—which involved someone outside the family—was taken out of my hands. I had agonised about this for a long time, fearful of what disclosure might do to two boys approaching puberty. At supper one night I was apologising for a recent bad patch, and explaining that I sometimes felt overwhelmed by the pain from my past, and my older son said out of the blue, 'Mum, were you sexually abused when you were young?' I started to cry, and agreed that I had been, and that it was an incredibly hard thing to have to cope with. The younger one jumped out of his chair and flung his arms round me and hugged me; the older one said how weird and horrible it must have been. Neither of them could understand why or how anyone could treat a child in this way; both of them recognised the reality of my pain.

The fact that they now knew my secret was a great relief to me, and seems not to have been a burden to them. On the contrary, they were glad to know why I was sometimes so sad—it helped them to understand that my moods and difficult behaviour were not the result of some fault in them, that they were not to blame. And as I've recovered they have learned a valuable lesson: that if you are suffering, you can find help; if you are wounded, you can heal.

Candida Hunt

◆

CONFRONTING THE PERPETRATOR

This is perhaps the hardest decision of all for survivors to make. It is probably best to be well advanced in your healing before you decide whether or not to confront your perpetrator. You must be unshakably sure of your own truth. You must be prepared for the perpetrator to use lies, denial, accusations of insanity or wickedness, manipulation—all the weapons at their disposal. You need to be reasonably confident that you will be able to stay in your adult self no matter what their reaction, and not revert to the child-state in which you were originally abused. You may have changed, but the perpetrator most likely will not have done, and will possibly attempt to re-exert their power in the old ways.

Many therapists in Australia advise clients against confronting the perpetrator, not so much because they feel it is inappropriate for the client but because they are afraid of the legal consequences for themselves. You cannot, therefore, necessarily count on your therapist to support you. But it is very important to have some reliable source of support before and immediately after the confrontation takes place: however well prepared you are, you will probably have some strong emotional reactions.

Some questions to ask when deciding whether to confront are: What do I hope to gain from this? Can I handle no reaction at all? Can I maintain my own reality in the face of total denial? Can I withstand the anger I am likely to face?

Let no one force you into confronting or not confronting. Part of regaining power and strength is finding the ability to make your own decisions on your own behalf. There is also no single right course of action to take when confronting. Some survivors prefer to write a letter; others to confront face to face. Some choose to be alone with the perpetrator, others to be accompanied by a trusted witness. Listen to advice from those you trust—and then make up your own mind about what to do and how to go about it.

I began to suspect I had been abused as long ago as 1983, but did not know for sure until mid-1986, when I had a single session of counselling in which I recalled oral abuse at two or three years of age. Later I read an article that contained a definition of abuse, and at that moment I *knew* I had been abused over a 20-year period.

By the end of 1987 I had enough recall to know the overall effect of the abuse, and had managed to move from the overriding fear I had of my father into anger. I felt it was right to confront my father. I had written to him in 1979, telling him I forgave him for 'everything', but not having a clue at that stage about the abuse. He had written back to say that saying thank you didn't seem adequate. I took his comment at face value at the time, but when I became aware of the abuse I realised the depth of meaning in his letter, and this gave me the courage to confront him. He acknowledged that he had indeed touched me inappropriately, and expressed his regret; this was important to me. His acknowledgement allowed me to begin to relate to him for the first time in my life. He and Mum visited me in 1989, and this occasion provided my only happy memories of Dad. When he died in 1991 my greatest grief was that there could be no more happy times with him.

Julie Waddy

◆

I would highly recommend that before confronting the perpetrator you have worked through the pain and abuse. It can be earth-shattering to receive the same treatment you got as a child, so you need to be very strong because when confronted they might try to use the same tactics to silence you again. If you are not prepared for it, it can just re-open old wounds. Don't expect them to admit that it happened, as it is only in very rare cases that this happens.

Not everyone needs to confront. I believe it is up to the individual. As a survivor it is always a temptation to try to protect your parents—but by protecting them you end up hurting yourself. It is always difficult to deal with feelings of love and hate towards your own parents, regardless of how violently and badly treated you were.

Linda Honey

◆

While I was having therapy I came to realise that something very private and sinister happened to me as a child that was too absurd to think about. It was behind a closed door. The words 'sexual abuse' pounded repeatedly through my mind. These words applied to someone else, not to me. The overwhelming shame of admitting my deepest fear finally gave way to the intense desire for truth. My father—it must have been my father, he was the only one close enough, the only one who would cause me to feel so unable to acknowledge the pain of reality that I would bury it deep in my subconscious.

Distrusting my 'woman's instinct', which hadn't worked too well in the past, I was driven to confront him. I placed an ISD call to my mother, who had been supportive up to a point, though the words 'psychiatrist' and 'therapy'—a slight on the family—had been a bitter pill for her to swallow. A supportive close family member wrote to my mother, forcing her to confront her own fears.

Several days later, the phone rang. On lifting the receiver I heard the familiar ISD beeps. 'Hallo,' I said, fearing the consequences.

'I'm sorry,' my father responded.

'What are you sorry for?' I asked. When he didn't answer, refusing to be robbed of my moment of freedom I pressed him: 'What are you sorry for, Dad?'

'I don't want to talk about it any more.' The phone went dead.

Feeling a sense of self-worth washing over me, I sat down and prayed. I wanted something more for all these years of torment . . . I wanted my freedom, God.

The next morning it came, the phone call I had been waiting for. 'Hallo,' I said over the familiar beeps.

'I did it,' said my father, 'I did it. I didn't mean to hurt you, I love you. I love you. I'm sorry,' he spluttered through tears of grief.

My knees went weak. Sobbing, I told him I forgave him, and all I wanted was to be set free from the secret, set free from the shame and guilt for something I had had no control over. I said, 'I know how much courage it has taken for you to confess the truth, Dad. I know how hard that can be.'

My dear mum had kept working on my dad all night until he finally broke down and admitted what he had done.

Rae

◆

There! I've told him and the earth hasn't swallowed me up—yet.

I finally focused on his face, which was one of shock and horror.

He then told me he didn't know, and I answered him by acknowledging that he may have been drunk—again.

Then he quietly asked me, 'You don't think that I knew what I was doing, do you?'

I told him that I would like to think that he was not consciously aware, but then again maybe he was aware, and that anyway it is beside the point. After all, his business 'liquid lunch' finished at 3.15 p.m., and he sexually abused me late at night. And what about the fact that I was only 12 and physically immature? My body was nothing like my mother's.

He became enraged at this afterthought of mine. How dare I suggest such a thing. 'Get out of my house!' he said. As I walked sadly to the door he told me that he was 'writing me off' as his daughter.

I stumbled back to my home (across the road), and then began a long and painful journey, fraught with self-doubt and guilt, that was to last two years. I was 37 years old.

My sisters and brother offered an initial attempt at support, and then quickly fell back into the safe dark place known as denial. I was soon regarded as the perpetrator and he the victim, as I had rocked the boat in a major way, and particularly as I had discussed the abuse with mutual friends.

My shining light through all of this was my husband, who was an unstinting source of support and empathy. He never tired of hearing my stories, nor did he recoil at the more unpleasant aspects. He was always available to comfort me on the bad days. There were also close friends who supported me, and continue to do so in the same loving way.

My mother suicided nine years ago, ignorant of my secret. I have withdrawn my relationship from my biological family as my father wants nothing more to do with me and has sought the protection and support of my siblings. It therefore made for a difficult and superficial association with his supporters, and I felt I had come too far to pretend any more that we were a happy unit. I now love myself unconditionally, and to continue in a relationship coloured by ongoing accusations and judgment would only undo my thriving healing process.

My confrontation with my father took place two years ago, and although it was extremely painful, I now live a happier life. I used to be so angry and rebellious, particularly with my husband. I know that he would never betray me as others have. I am also able to forgive my siblings, as I understand that they have their own journey of enlightenment and truth to seek, and that their choice may be important to that process. I forgave my father a long time ago, probably because I pity him and feel sad at the prospect that he will die reflecting on the suffering he has inflicted on others.

Susan Pratt

◆

As a ritual abuse survivor I have many perpetrators to confront, in the immediate family as well as in the cult.

My father was the hardest hurdle to overcome. As controller and manipulator he would set it up so that my mum looked like the bad person. I had to see the lies and confront him. This I did through many means—direct confrontation when I was 16, telling him off in the street, hanging up the phone on him, etc. The latest was to write to him listing all the abuse that he has inflicted on me and my family. I felt free then. It was all there, and I had said all that I wanted to say. Once I could do that, I was able to confront the cult.

The media is the best avenue to do this. Cults thrive on secrecy. I have been on national television, have written for a student newspaper, have been on ABC regional radio, been in the local newspaper encouraging people to testify before the NSW Royal Commission into police corruption. Every time I go public, I feel more real. Each time I feel that another survivor will respond and feel validated, that society will begin to understand the truth, as they have with incest and domestic violence. With each survivor who escapes we will unravel another knot in the tangle.

John David

◆

For those of you with recovered memories who would like to confront but fear denial, I can tell you that denial from abusers can be just as vehement even when you've always remembered.

I have never forgotten the severe batterings my mother gave me as a child. When I was four she held my head under water in the bath. Later came black eyes, bloody noses, tufts of hair torn out of my head. She would throw me to the floor and repeatedly stamp on my stomach, drag me along by the hair, kicking my body as she went. My mother pulled a knife on me when I was 13. Shortly after this, I decided I'd have to fight back. Terribly vicious scenes ensued throughout my teens. Yet when I was 20 and confronted her about the childhood bashings, her response was: 'You evil little liar'. She still tells people I am mad.

I also confronted by letter the person who raped me when I was 14. I wrote and re-wrote the letter till it said what I felt I wanted it to. My feelings afterwards were initially sad, as if that dear 14-year-old inside me could not believe someone would actually stand up for her. I was also afraid of his power, of standing up to him. What if I angered him and he hurt me again?

However, when these feelings faded I felt immensely strong, and I still do. I think it is a powerful thing to do, and for me definitely worthwhile, but I would say *never* to push yourself.

As for the perpetrator whose abuses I repressed, I still feel unready to confront here, but that's OK, I'll go with my own process and see what happens.

I think it is important to confront very much for yourself, with no expectations of receiving anything from the perpetrator.

Louise Plummer

◆

My father was too violent and angry for me ever to engage in a proper confrontation with him. I would try and talk to my mother, but she continually defended both her and my father's actions. (Anyway, I 'deserved' everything I got; they were my parents, so 'You obey us' continued to be the rule.) About three years after my father died I invited Mother to stay with us in Sydney. My attempt to begin a dialogue about my abuse was met with denial, accusations, defensiveness and attempted justification.

The most frustrating aspect was feeling that I just didn't get through to her in any way—that she was still stuck on her own planet and had no idea where I was coming from. I'd built up hope that she'd changed as a person, had maybe 'reinvented' herself as a widow, as many women do. I thought she'd be more open to admitting some major mistakes on her and my father's part. I was hoping she would validate my feelings and experiences, and maybe reveal what was really going through their minds when they were abusing me. Hoping to bridge the gap between us, I planned to ask about her relationship with her own father, which she was also reluctant to talk about. This was something my parents felt children had no right to know—it was only their business. But to me it was part of my background, and very much my business too.

With my mother, nothing had changed. My disappointment at the outcome of that visit was on many levels.

About two months later I started having severe mental difficulties. When people spoke to me I'd feel no connection between who they thought they were talking to and who I thought I was. I felt split in half emotionally, and seemed to see everything as if through a long tunnel. I also came to hate myself, to the point where I wished I could walk out of a room and leave myself behind in it. I am convinced this was due largely to the non-event of Mother's visit. We had spoken on the phone a few times since then, but always ended up arguing. I had to face the fact that while I had grown and thought and felt differently and more deeply about things, she was stuck in the same old pattern and refused to change because it was nice and safe where she was, and she could live more happily in denial. I was angry that I had made such an effort to reconcile things—without blaming or accusation, just trying to discuss the facts—and she didn't want to know, and refused to acknowledge anything I was trying to achieve.

Jacqueline Frajer

✦

I was sexually abused by my stepfather. He married my mother four months after my fourth birthday. He had already entered my vagina with his finger, and the assaults continued spasmodically until I was 22 years old. In desperation I confided in my GP, who said that by confronting him I would make it stop. Somehow I found the courage to confront my tormentor.

This is what happened. I found out that my mother had known—not the extent or the frequency of the abuse, but that I had been abused, and had done nothing. The family couldn't cope. I felt alone and unloved. Eventually everything settled into a semblance of normality, and it was never mentioned again. The abuse did stop, but the legacy lived on.

Finally, at 37 years of age, after an abusive marriage and years of counselling, I have learned to face the effects and begin a journey to the real me. However, I have never forgotten, and when I saw the isolating of my three-year-old niece and recognised the 'grooming process' begin again, the horrors returned.

This time I was stronger, and able to face the fear. I again confronted my stepfather and also my sister with my experience and my suspicions. My need to protect my nieces overcame my conditioning to 'keep it secret'. Even so, it took me several months of soul-searching and the support of my counsellor to reach the decision to speak out.

Would I be ostracised? What if I was wrong? Self-doubt and fear plagued my mind. In the end it all spilled out unrehearsed when my sister told me over the phone that my niece had been taken out in the car by our stepfather. It had often been the setting for my own abuse, and I found myself revisiting my childhood traumas as I shared my concerns with my sister.

I'd love to be able to say that everything worked out well.

For my nieces, hopefully, it has. The secret has once again been broken. My mother and stepfather minimised my abuse, and then decided to tell everyone that I had been lying. They decreed that I was no longer part of the family, and was not to be informed of family events. (The family live in Scotland, and I am in Australia.) I missed my aunt's funeral and my mother's serious illness and hospitalisation, and had no contact from the family. It was a painful time.

I don't know what the future holds, but I know that by confronting the abuse and my abuser the secrecy has ended. My nieces are hopefully safe to enjoy the childhood that was denied me, and I am at last free.

Gillian Graham

◆

I thought the confrontation would give me release, but it just made me angry all over again. I gave him an opportunity to say sorry, or even just acknowledge his actions; he said he had been foolish— *foolish*! Not good enough. I also did not get support from my family. They prefer the status quo, not the truth. There was definite merit in laying the blame squarely where it belongs instead of feeling guilty—that was empowering—and also to stop punishing my partner just for being a man. It was not, however, a life-changing experience. There was no joyous forgiving or loving, just continuing to live and struggling to be me—every day.

It took another two years before I could speak out about the incest to my father again. I said this: 'For years I kept hoping you would do or say something to indicate that you were responsible for what happened, and that this would somehow ease the terrible guilt I felt. I now accept that this will never happen, you don't have the courage or strength to do this. But that doesn't mean I have to be guilty. I am an adult now, and am in control of my life. I am not a child any more, the child too afraid to run away and too scared to stay. It's not now, and never was, my secret.'

Nothing changed, but I felt stronger.

Wendy Stamp

✦

There came a time in my healing when I just knew that the time had come to confront Jack. When I had made the decision to do this, I felt panic-stricken. I was truly petrified. I knew I needed to be well prepared, so I thought about what I could do to minimise my fear of seeing him and my therapist and I role-played several confrontations. I made a list of all the possible reactions Jack might have.

He could deny it, say it never happened. He could be angry, he could be violent. He could say it was my fault—that I'd made him do it. He could be sad. He might not remember it. He could say that my therapist planted the memories. He could be scared at having to face the reality he's denied his entire life. He might be afraid of what I might do—if I was going to take him to court or call his wife or something. He could get defensive. He might simply get up and leave. He might threaten me. He might call me a liar. He might threaten my family if I tell anyone else. He might say that he can see how that's what I believe. He might admit it. He might cry. He might tell me things about himself to try and make me feel sorry for him.

I practised what I was going to say. I had a mental picture of how I wanted the confrontation to be. I knew that I wanted my best friend to be there to give me courage and strength.

I got to the restaurant early on Saturday, and Rhonda and I sat down to wait. It's hard to put into words how I was feeling. The anxiety was brutal. My stomach was so badly twisted in knots I was having some difficulty breathing. The waiting was the hardest part.

Finally, Jack arrived. When I saw him I felt myself tighten up and relax at the same time. The moment had finally come, and I suddenly became calm. After exchanging stiff, meaningless pleasantries, I told him why I had summoned him. Sitting across that table from him, I was so glad about all my preparation. I found myself able to respond well to anything he said. He had many reactions—most of the responses I had included on my potential reaction list did actually take place.

I had decided to tape the confrontation. It is difficult to hear what Jack was saying, but the tape picked up my voice fairly well. I didn't tell Jack about the tape recorder; I wanted to have a record of the conversation for myself. I knew I'd be so anxious and nervous that I wouldn't be able to remember what I'd said and done. It is important to me that I have this record, and it made it much easier to recount the confrontation to other people. Here are some extracts of what I said.

'My job, my goal here isn't to convince you so that you would say, "Yes, I remember, I did it, I'm sorry". That's not what I'm looking for. What I'm looking for is just to tell you, to see you face to face . . .

'Whether you remember or you don't frankly isn't my concern. But part of my healing process, after being shut up about it for twenty-three years, is to open my mouth and to say, "This is what happened". And it's not going to happen to me ever again . . .

'I'll tell you what, Jack. For twenty-three years I had no recollection of it, so it actually doesn't surprise me that you can't remember it now. Because it's kind of a heinous thing, it's not the easiest thing to remember. And believe me, when I started having the memories, it was incredibly painful and incredibly difficult and I didn't want to believe it. It may come back to you in a while like it came back to me; it may—or it may not. Frankly, Jack, it doesn't matter either way. It doesn't matter to me if it comes back to you because I know it happened. I didn't imagine it, I know it's true, and there's nothing in the world you can say that would convince me otherwise.'

However he tried to steer the conversation, I was ready. I became stronger and more powerful as time want on. When I had said everything I wanted to say, I got up and walked out.

I was really pleased with how well I had done. I don't mean to sound arrogant; I just feel it is important to be proud of myself. I spent so many years feeling useless and inferior, it's an important gift to myself to be proud of myself and my actions.

I think one thing that affected the confrontation was that I knew exactly what I wanted, and it was not dependent on his reaction. I only wanted him to know that I'd remembered. I just needed to tell him that. I had absolutely nothing invested in his response; it truly didn't matter to me. I never needed him to acknowledge the truth, or to say, 'I'm so sorry'. That wasn't the point.

When I walked out of the restaurant after confronting him I found I had healed the vast majority of the damage he had done to me. What happens to me now, sometimes, is that something may happen that triggers me back to the feelings I had then, or to something that took place then. Some of the effects of the rape are still with me: I may have a reaction that is a huge overreaction to an incident occurring now, and I know it is based on what Jack did to me. So I am not yet completely healed of the effects of having been raped. But for me confrontation was a huge step, a huge closure in my healing process.

Karen I. Shanbrom

◆

I had been on a spiritual journey of healing and discovery for almost five years when the time came for me to think about confrontation. I felt I had gone past the feelings of wanting revenge, answers, apologies or validation of my abuse. I simply *needed* to confront. I had prayed for the strength to forgive my abuser, and although I didn't feel as though I could, I made an act of will, and left the rest to God. I was still angry, but I felt the anger towards my abuser had subsided enough to allow me a positive experience. I believe anger to be a positive emotion, and there are ways of expressing it that foster a sense of empowerment and triumph. With the support of my sister, I confronted my perpetrator, telling my story with conviction, power and sorrow over my lost innocence. He could hardly remember, having been an alcoholic at the time, but he was so shocked and dismayed that he remained speechless for some time. He then apologised, not only for the terrible injustice of the abuse itself, but for the fact that I had lived the next 20 years in emotional hell, bitter towards my whole family, scarred beyond belief.

I could not have asked for a more sincere response, though I believe I was very lucky. He was finally able to fit the pieces of his unhappy life together, and take on responsibility for his actions and their repercussions. I felt the huge weight of secrecy lifting as I drove away.

This was a huge turning point in my recovery, and I thank God for his strength in enabling me to face the source of my anguish, and look towards my future, full of hope and liberty.

Melinda Witt

◆

GOING PUBLIC

The only way any of us can help to prevent abuse is to speak out, to let people hear our story and understand our pain. Until recently the only people talking on behalf of survivors were the professionals. Reports and statistics are better than nothing, but our truth is far more telling. In the press there have also been numerous stories about how child abuse does not affect you as an adult, how children are naturally promiscuous, and other nonsensical things. These as well as the false memory myth were allowed to gain credence because we had not found our own voice, the courage to stand up and say, 'What rubbish!', and to speak out about the effects abuse has had on us throughout our lives. As we heal, if we possibly can we must speak out. We alone know the truth, and it is up to us to tell it. It is difficult, it is wearing, but it helps more than anything else we can do to break the taboo, the silence that has allowed child abuse to flourish in Australia.

We applaud the courage of our contributors who have spoken publicly.

I recovered my first memories of abuse approximately four years ago. These memories had been repressed for more than 40 years. What unfolded was the knowledge that my father had abused me sexually, physically and emotionally for most of my childhood. What also became clear, to my great horror, was that he had similarly abused my two eldest children when I left them in their grandparents' care.

For the last seven years I have been working as a psychologist in private practice in central Victoria. When I worked with clients who had been abused—and it did seem that I had some invisible sign outside that said, 'Come this way all who have been abused'!—I was moved by their courage. I often wondered how I would deal with such an experience as theirs, at the time not realising that my own past was similar to that of some of my clients.

As I began my own recovery process, I was faced with an inner conflict. The professional part of me wanted to gain and increase peer acceptance, and develop a professional reputation for good work; I also needed to provide for my children. Another part of me, the survivor, was not prepared to remain silent any longer. The survivor part wanted to tell her story, to be heard—and especially by those with power and influence.

By a slow process, and with the encouragement of other courageous survivors who were prepared to speak out publicly, I gradually negotiated an agreement between these two parts of myself. The survivor part would be allowed to speak to the professional part's peers, provided that the survivor didn't 'lose the plot' and become emotionally charged. The professional part could run the show, as long as she didn't deny what the survivor part was feeling, and allowed her to tell her story.

An opportunity presented itself where I had the chance to speak to my peers about the abuse I had experienced. For weeks before-hand my fear and anxiety made me wonder whether I would get a word out. I knew it was important to put in place all the support I could gather—from friends, my partner and other professionals.

The time came to speak, and to my amazement I had little or no anxiety. I felt clear and strong, and that was how I addressed the audience. What occurred, I believe, was a moment of true healing: the process of integration, the opposite of the disintegration that was part of the terrible damage done so long ago.

The audience was responsive and empathic, and some people were deeply moved by my story. They were generous in their feed-back. I hoped that at least one professional would come to under-stand what the experience of being a survivor was like. A more ambitious hope was that by speaking out myself I might encourage other professionals who have been abused to speak out too. My ultimate aim was to cut through the feelings of shame, the need to hide this ghastly mess, and by so doing help to force society to see what it would prefer not to see.

The worst abuse is often carried out in the most 'respectable' homes, in families where abusers are intelligent, professional and well-respected citizens in the community. What these perpetrators do not take into account is that their children will also become professionals—interestingly, often in areas such as psychology—which may help them not only with their past experience, but also to speak out about it in influential quarters where other survivors might not have the opportunity to talk.

At the time of writing this, I am being faced yet again with the horrors of the past, this time in relation to one of my children. This is probably the ultimate pain for me, and fills me with the utmost outrage. It gives me all the more reason to believe that we must speak out on behalf of those who have been abused, who are being abused, and who are vulnerable to abuse.

Marie E. O'Neill

If there is one thing that this whole ordeal has taught me or enabled me to understand, it is that I am worth every single bit of it. I am worth fighting tooth and nail for, and I am proud to write letters voicing concern about the legal system and its apparent direction. I am also proud to say I won't back down.

He abused me and what he did was wrong. I count. I am important. I am a unique, beautiful creation of God. What happened to me should *not* have happened, and as long as he's alive he's going to know it!

We are survivors. We each have the strength within. It keeps us alive—it keeps us fighting—fighting for the truth, and fighting to make sure that it won't happen again.

Chris Lord

I made an important decision, one that I knew would change my life, though to what extent I could not know at the time. I had a number of reasons for deciding to speak to the media: first, my own desire to reach out to other survivors, to let them know that they were not alone; second, I felt emotionally strong enough at the time to do it; and third, I found a reporter I felt I could trust.

During the interview I felt a strong sense of empowerment, and once the article was published a great sense of relief in knowing that I had done what I had wanted to do. The response I have received because of the article has been overwhelming. A support group has been established, and I have been offered the services of a counsellor for the group. A number of other survivors have been able to break the silence of their own abuse as a result of reading the article. I have been approached by one of the local state high schools about formulating a child abuse prevention programme to be implemented as part of the school curriculum. I have received many phone calls and letters from other survivors.

For me personally, there has been an emotional backlash in the stirring up of memories and feelings about my abuse, but I knew there would be. That is the price I paid to do what I felt needed to be done, and I have no regrets, not one. My story of my own abuse was a gift to other survivors—a gift I was happy to give.

I will not let what was done to me in the past stop me from doing what I want to do in my life now. I will not let it beat me. I will not let it win. I will continue to work to help other survivors and to protect children now from being abused because I know it is the right thing to do, not just for other people but also for myself.

If I can help to bring other survivors in from the cold as others have helped me through my own journey, then that is reward enough. Telling my own story of abuse to the media has been a major step in my own healing process, and all in all it has been both extremely rewarding and empowering.

Mary Abraham

◆

My story is now being investigated by the police. I reached a point where if there was no confrontation of the truth, I didn't know how I could continue.

David Patterson

◆

My reasons for going to court and revealing my abuse were many. As those readers who have been abused or read to this point will know, guilt and shame are two of the major consequences of sexual abuse or indeed any other form of victimisation. Shame in particular requires and feeds off silence. The best antidote for shame is breaking the wall of secrecy that surrounds the abuse and its consequences. The clearer the victim of abuse becomes about the real nature of what happened and the proper location for blame and guilt, the more able he is to reveal his secret. This reduces the shame. Practice makes perfect, so the more times the secrecy is broken, and the wider the audience the victim addresses, the more potentially effective this process can be in lessening shame and promoting recovery.

It is difficult enough to tell those who love us. It is harder to tell less intimate acquaintances. Most difficult of all is being prepared to deal effectively with those who respond by blaming the victim for what happened. In going through the court process, there are many opportunities for coming out and breaking the secrecy and shame.

Going to court required me to focus on particular points and become clear about them in preparation for the cross-examination. In my case, the topics I was most anxious about were those on which I had judged myself most harshly. Concern that one may be a homosexual is an important issue for men who have been sexually abused in childhood by men, and this is a common target for attack by the perpetrator's barrister, who will attempt to distort your testimony.

People everywhere have a powerful need for justice and fairness, for the appropriate labelling of right and wrong. Accompanying this are legitimate desires to see the perpetrators of injustice punished and made to pay for their behaviour. I also needed to stop him from continuing to offend, on the assumption that most perpetrators continue to do so. Even if the outcome of the trial is a 'not guilty' verdict, the perpetrator may think twice about offending again.

Finally, the entire procedure validated my experience. The seriousness with which our society and its courts treat this crime helped me to see more clearly the true nature of the events of my childhood. I felt that I was contributing to the exposure of the prevalence of childhood sexual abuse in our society, and to the process of declaring this unacceptable to current and future perpetrators.

Peter West

◆

I was able to be clear about who the real perpetrator was, and to separate emotionally from the abuse. Going to the police, and sending the information that I had done so back to him, made me more safe. The NSW Royal Commission into the police service was also important. Here was a place that was open to my evidence. The people were really supportive. I felt that I had actually freed myself from the burden of knowing all this horrendous and extremely criminal stuff. Knowing that there are other survivors doing the same has meant that my evidence will be supported. We got the evidence out.

John David

◆

The fact that he had to front up at the trial felt very empowering to me. It showed him that I hadn't forgotten what he did to me, that he was responsible and accountable for his actions, that it wasn't my fault, but his.

Olivia-Mai Ryan

◆

I did it to break his control over me, and to show that his threats of killing me if I ever spoke about the abuse were no longer effective. I also broke the conspiracy of silence by forcing a courtroom to listen to everything about my abuse. Although my father was acquitted, I still felt it was a positive experience for me. I felt empowered by what I had done. I stood up to him and forced him to make himself accountable.

Penny Stevens

◆

In 1994, my counselling came to the point where I had to decide what I was going to do about the perpetrators. Was it enough that they seemed to be able to slide into the background and pretend it never happened? Was I content with the knowledge that I had never really received an apology or acknowledgement from them, that what they did to me was absolutely filthy, evil and wrong? The answer I found coming to me more and loudly each time I thought about it was NO—it wasn't OK. For once I was accepting the fact that I was more important than they were, and it was not OK for it to be just quietly dealt with behind closed doors.

Coming out for me involved my father finally knowing what happened, and sending off letters to the perpetrators. My counsellor had already told me of the difficulty that I might encounter with the police, but I think I was somewhat blinded at first by the fact that I admired them so much for their efforts against crime, and also for the fact that I was the victim in all this so I believed I would be helped.

Two years later one of the perpetrators has been jailed, and the other may avoid the courts because of his age, which I find very difficult to accept. However, I do still feel the experience has been worthwhile.

Chris Lord

◆

Layne (not her real name) stepped up to the witness stand in the District Court. She was there to describe to the 12 strangers sitting before her in the jury box what her stepfather had done to her. Over the next several hours, she gave details of the times and places where the digital penetration, oral sex and attempted penile penetration had occurred.

Layne's stepfather sexually assaulted her for more than six years, from the time she was eight. The man also abused her sister and, at one stage, raped a 12-year-old friend staying in their house.

It was not until she was in her late 20s that Layne felt strong enough to report the assault to police. She had told her mother years earlier but was not believed. Eventually, her stepfather faced more than a dozen charges.

'I was really afraid because I had seen in movies the things that lawyers do,' Layne says. 'I was a bit intimidated by [the stepfather] being in the room but not as intimidated as I was by the defence barrister. That was the most traumatic part of the whole thing, the defence barrister. He was ridiculing the whole thing, making jokes about it.'

Her stepfather's barrister quizzed her extensively about her boyfriends and her sex life in the years after the attacks. He even asked about a schoolteacher who had supported her at one stage in her life, implying some inappropriate relationship.

'It was all the attention to irrelevant detail that got me. He would ask where did you go after the attack in the back yard, and where after that. I felt the whole way through that it was about me absolutely proving it, which I know is what you have to do, but it was a matter of my credibility . . .'

Layne's stepfather was found guilty on six counts and pleaded guilty to another four. He was sentenced to a minimum of four years jail. Layne thinks the sentence was too lenient but is pragmatic enough to know that every victim would probably feel the same way.

Like many victims of child sexual assault, she was not able to come forward until adulthood—until, as she says, 'I felt strong and felt it was the right time in my life to let him know he couldn't get away with it, that he had to be punished.'

It was undoubtedly one of the most difficult things she has ever done but, when asked if she would go through it all again, she answers, 'yep' without hesitating. 'I think at the time I felt drained and belittled. But with hindsight, I am not as embarrassed and I feel empowered.'

Jennie Curtin, reporting in the Sydney Morning Herald

◆

My Saturday night Bible reading was Ezekiel 2: 'Stand on your feet, speak out to a rebellious nation. Some will listen, others don't want to.' During that night, I didn't get very much sleep; the words filled my head: 'Stand up in My house and speak.'

So I went off to church on Sunday morning with my husband Bob for the 8 a.m. service. Near the end of the service, during prayers for the sick and troubled, our minister stopped. All were silent. No one else had prayed at any of the prayer sections. I stood up in the aisle, my back to the door, and spoke.

'I am standing here, Father, as you told me to stand. My daughter came to this church for help about being sexually abused. She was given no help. My husband and I asked for help, and were given none. We were told not to tell anyone in the church about it. There was a young lass in the church who had her innocence taken from her and who was then lied and talked about in the church. No one helped her, and she has left the church.

'There are sexually abused people within the church fearful of speaking out, made to feel second-class Christians. You, Father, want them to be cared for, helped and listened to; to be held and comforted, not condemned. Not to have guilt placed upon them because they could not live up to ideas of the people who did not want to understand. All you are asking is for your people to understand, to help them, to listen to them, to care for them and not turn away from them. Holy Father, I praise you for the love of Jesus. And Lord, I am standing here alone.'

When I had finished the church was quiet. I could hear muted crying. The silence seemed never ending. Then the minister began the prayers for Communion. A woman came up to me still crying, hugged me and said, 'It had to be done, thank you'. After the service finished they came, mostly women, hugging me, a few still in tears. The same words, 'It had to be said', 'I will tell you now of women I know about who are suffering'. Some people couldn't get past me quick enough, but others—including men—stopped to say something on their way out. The minister came and hugged me and said, 'I never knew, why didn't you tell me?' (I had told our other minister.)

On Tuesday night the phone call came from our minister. We talked and talked about our pain, then he told me of his own family and their pain. Yes, sexual abuse. I had spoken out, and he was then able to share the horror of his own family. Doing what I did made it possible for others to speak about their own pain. We are not alone. I am still being told of people in our church who are suffering: the door has been opened, the pain is being exposed, and now there is a chance for healing.

The shame is not ours to carry. The burden belongs to those who committed the crime against us as children. We must keep the doors open so that others can feel safe enough to come forward and speak out.

Pat Wagstaff

◆

I AM WALKING
I am walking the road less travelled
trying to find the real me
my soul wanting to be free from oppression
I now speak the truth and set my soul free.

Linda Honey

CHAPTER SIX

✦

Healing

We are healed by what we turn towards, not what we turn from.
Allegra Taylor, *Older Than Time*

The Macquarie Dictionary defines the word heal as: To make whole or sound; to restore to health; to make free from ailment or to free from anything evil or distressing. To cleanse or purify.

Doesn't that sound wonderful? Does it sound unrealistic? When we are bound up in our pain, caged in the dark pit of depression, angry beyond belief or full of guilt and despair, it can seem quite impossible that we should ever feel differently. But we can change. We can all change. The fact that we have survived against terrible odds is proof of our capacity for learning, for growth, for self-protection, for adapting to new and difficult circumstances—and above all, as we have said before, it is proof of our courage. All these qualities are at our service in the quest for healing. It is as natural for humans to want to grow and heal as it is for plants to turn towards the light. In a way, that is what we are doing when we acknowledge our pain, recognise our urge to heal, and take our first steps in the healing journey.

The speed with which the painful symptoms of past abuses present themselves to be dealt with will depend upon many things: how strong you are, what else is happening in your life, the extent of the abuse and how you internalised it in the first place, how much loving support you can count on. Working your way through the symptoms, the memories and the feelings is often like peeling an onion—each new layer brings tears to your eyes, and the removal of each layer brings you closer to the heart of the hurt child.

Survivors often want to know, 'How long will it take? When will I be healed?' No one can tell. It will happen in its own time—it is already happening. You have started on the journey by reading this book. Like the growth of a child's body, it happens little by little each day, though you may not be aware of it. Whether you are awake or asleep, laughing, crying or working your way through a period of anxiety, you are still in the process of healing. And again like the child's body, sometimes there are growth spurts, when you make rapid progress, and at other times growth slows down, while you adjust to the changes that are taking place.

One important stage in the healing process is relearning how to trust. Children are born trusting. No one teaches them this, they just arrive in the world ready to rely on and trust those whose task it is to protect them. If that trust is misused and abused, the child wisely stops trusting. This life-saving lesson may later prevent survivors from being able to discriminate between who is trustworthy and who is not. We have included a whole section on survivors' experiences of therapy; when you are feeling vulnerable it is not easy to have the courage of your convictions, and to distinguish a helpful therapist from a damaging one. Finding a trustworthy therapist is an important step in healing.

It's not just other people that you need to learn to trust. At the time of the abuse, many children shut down some of their physical senses and emotional responses in an effort not to feel what is happening to them. The effect of this is that we can no longer rely on our own senses to guide us in the choices we make and the way we conduct our lives. We need to learn to trust ourselves again, too, and as we heal, we will.

Just as every aspect of our lives has in some way been affected by the abuse, so too does the healing gradually seep into everything we are and everything we do. We may have been working on one set of issues, and suddenly realise that something else—the way we relate to someone, doing something kind for ourselves, saying no without feeling guilty—has also become possible. Many people find that a spiritual dimension to their life emerges during the healing process, and that contributes to what is often a real transformation. As we begin to heal, we discover feelings such as love, happiness, joy and wonder that seem little short of miraculous. This miracle is a natural one: we were intended all along to know joy as well as suffering, love as well as pain.

If you are at the beginning of your healing journey, we hope that the stories in this chapter will inspire you and bring you hope, and that the time will soon come when you can celebrate your own healing and find your own joy.

THERAPISTS

The question the staff at ASCA are most often asked is, 'How can I find a good therapist?' Sadly, it is not an easy question to answer. There are not very many high-quality therapists around, and very few who are affordable. Some people working in psychology and psychiatry are wise, empathic and compassionate; some are not. If you find a helpful therapist the first time you are lucky; it often takes determination and extraordinary persistence to keep searching if you have bad experiences with the people who are meant to be helping you. Seek advice from other survivors, the sexual assault services, or ASCA.

How can you tell if your therapist is any good? You will start to feel better immediately. There will be challenging times ahead, but if you feel safe with them, respected by them, you will eventually learn to trust them. If a therapist abuses that trust, it is enormously damaging—and as the accounts in this section show, this does happen. Do not feel that because you are the client or the patient, you have no power and no rights. Therapy is a partnership, and you have the right to evaluate whether the therapist is a benign or malign influence on your healing.

At ASCA we have a list of therapists who work in this area and whose work we respect.

At present I am faced with a dilemma I think survivors must often face. I wish to know more to enable me to become whole and fully alive, but I am afraid of what it will be like if I recover more memories. How traumatic will it be? Will it disrupt my relationship with a partner who provides me with a fulfilling and loving relationship? How will I cope as a mother and breadwinner?

I want both to know more, and to put it all behind me and get on with my life. Is it possible to do both—to work through the trauma and stay functional? I believe it is possible if the therapist is chosen carefully. I also know that at some level I do not have a choice—my past is continually in my present, and when I try to ignore my abused child, she comes to the fore, frequently inappropriately, and creates havoc. This leads me to the question of what I consider to be important criteria in selecting a therapist to work with recovering my memories.

The prime need is to feel safe and to feel heard. Unless the 'abused child' part of me feels safe and reassured, the process will not happen. Safety means a therapist who is predictable, who can bear to hear my story, who can survive and not react to my intense feelings, and who can stay with me in a non-judgmental and accepting way as I explore my past. Only in such an environment will I begin to trust the working alliance and the therapist's need at times to confront, to challenge me, or to stay with his/her difference.

My second need is to know that the therapist will not collude with my unconscious denial, that is, my need at times to deny or minimise or reframe the past. The memories and perceptions I am recovering are valid, and it is important that I do not give them up, lose them or bury them as I did in the past. Contrary to the idea that therapists are planting false memories in their clients' minds, I believe what happens more frequently is that clients resist recovering their memories until such time as they are able to bear the knowledge. Where incest is involved, the client needs the therapist's help to face the fact that someone you loved, trusted and depended on was the one who did you such harm. This is very difficult to believe and accept, even in the face of considerable evidence. It can take years of therapy to become able to accept the truth about the abuse.

My third need is for what I would call a 'strong' therapist. It is the 'stronger' survivors who are able to tolerate knowing they were abused and are able to come to therapy. These clients have large amounts of what I call 'psychic energy', and need therapists who are able to tolerate their intense feelings within the therapeutic relationship. Such clients constantly 'push' the therapist to test his or her limits and strength; it can be quite a challenge for a therapist to survive the survivor.

Marie E. O'Neill

◆

Here are my suggestions about the therapist's role. They should:
- provide a safe environment
- listen to and hear clients and validate their experience, not give advice, direct or lead clients, or act as a detective
- see the client as the expert in his or her own life
- respect clients and their experience
- allow clients to recount their experience at their own pace, and help them make sense of their experience, not elicit memories
- offer unconditional positive regard, and accept the client as a fellow human being
- provide client-centred, not therapist-centred, therapy.

Ester Miro

◆

I was so lucky to have a wonderful psychologist who believed in the use of hypnosis. Much has been written and claimed against hypnosis, but I would never have recovered my memories without it—or rather, I would have done but only after many more years in treatment. I was totally conscious while being hypnotised. It is not the sort of hypnosis that we see on television. The therapist does not intrude. I remember absolutely everything about it, including the rather strange sensation that while I was recounting what had happened to me as a child, in a childlike voice, and while I was feeling all the emotions associated with those events, my adult self was watching, observing, and in a sense learning from my own child about my pain. Hypnosis took down my 'sensible', 'controlling' self and allowed my child to be heard.

I think this sort of work is so different from what we all think of as hypnosis that it should be given another name—perhaps 'reliving'. What I experienced while 'reliving' was absolutely clear, and quite different from the usual experience of remembering. Now I have relived these parts of my childhood, they are in my ordinary memory and are liable to the normal process of forgetfulness. I would recommend hypnosis to anyone—as long as it is done with a therapist who is trustworthy and professional— particularly if you are like me, with very strong and well-developed defence mechanisms that in my normal conscious state are almost impossible to break down.

Liz Mullinar

◆

My experience with therapists has been mixed. Over a period of 17 years I saw GPs, psychiatrists, a psychologist, a member of a mental health team, members of the clergy and natural therapists. Because I had suppressed the memories of sexual abuse, I was not able to say, 'I was sexually abused when I was a child and I need help'. I was displaying symptoms of post-traumatic stress and describing dissociation (without realising it myself), but I was never asked any questions about my childhood.

From my experience, it seems that people in the medical profession have not been trained to recognise the signs of childhood abuse in adults, and their understanding and knowledge of the severe long-term damage that abuse causes sometimes leaves a lot to be desired. However, when I did start remembering my abuse it was seeing a psychiatrist (half of whose practice was with survivors) and staying in a hospital where the staff were aware and understood the after-effects of child abuse. That had a positive effect on my healing.

I would look for a therapist/counsellor who knows and understands the effects of abuse. Thankfully I found such a counsellor, who is herself a survivor. She works with the local sexual assault service, and for seven years also ran a therapy group. She was respectful, and saw herself not as the healer but as one who gives clients the tools they need to face the pain that is part of the healing process. She did a wonderful job, showing much care and giving a great deal of support, thus empowering her clients in a healthy way.

Since dealing with my abuse I have seen a GP who was very understanding and allowed me to talk and cry. She respected my pain without wanting just to medicate me, which had happened to me before. I have also recently seen a GP who has patients fill out a questionnaire about their past, as he recognises the fact that any unresolved childhood trauma can affect us in adulthood, and also considers the strong link between our emotions and our physical body, realising that emotional damage often shows itself in a physical way.

I believe also that the clergy need more education, because in many cases people go to them with problems which may have childhood abuse as the underlying cause, and unless the pastor, minister or priest is trained to recognise possible abuse their help is not very effective.

Maureen Searson

◆

I became immobilised many times, unable even to care for myself adequately as the pain was just overwhelming. I now realise how important it is to seek help. I don't think it is something you can do on your own, as healing comes from reaching out.

As a child I was helpless, but as an adult I came to realise that I was responsible for doing something about it. I have been to three therapists in my search for someone really skilled in dealing with sexual abuse. I was fortunate to find the therapist I have now, who has done a lot of work on herself and has dealt with much of her own pain so she is able to be there for me and help me work through mine.

In order to heal I had to face and deal with my pain and anguish, which I was unable to do on my own. My counsellor would pick up when I was taking refuge by staying 'in my head', and helped me to face my feelings, teaching me that in order to heal I needed to feel what was really going on inside me and not analyse things. Be careful of any counsellors who try to get you simply to work it through in your head. This was where I lived most of my life; I was a master at thinking everything through, but it isn't the answer.

It takes a great deal of courage to seek professional help. I had been trying to do it on my own but my untreated issues were never dealt with and it wasn't until I found someone who had training and worked with sexual abuse that I learned to feel safe. My counsellor also understood and worked with inner child issues, which helped me integrate and heal.

When looking for a good counsellor, find out if they have worked on their own issues. Unfortunately, many of them haven't, and they can do more harm than good. You need to feel safe and trust the therapist's ability to handle rage, anger, grief and sadness, and to be sensitive to your fears. A really good therapist is one who is intuitive to your needs and feelings, not relying only on logic, and can help you to find your own answers, which empowers you.

The worst experience I had was with my first therapist. She helped me build my self-confidence, which was good, but she defended my mother, trying to imply that she really couldn't have known what was happening. This invalidated my truth, my whole reality. She seemed incapable of handling my anger, which was directed at my mother for knowing but not doing anything to stop it. I felt so let down and betrayed again, and I didn't want her telling me what 'really' happened. She had no way of knowing, as she hadn't lived through the experience—and I had!

Linda Honey

◆

Therapy seems to take a lot of forms, with all sorts of ideas. Sometimes it has helped, sometimes it hasn't. Sometimes it has torn me to pieces.

My first introduction to it was at the age of 23, when I went for help about my drinking and my father's drinking. At the time, I also mentioned the sexual abuse by Grandpa when I was six years old. Despite my drinking, it was on my mind. The woman's response was, 'Oh, you probably felt guilty about enjoying yourself. Why don't you read a book on women's sexual fantasies?' I had no idea at the time how inadequate this response was.

My next venture for help was to see a 'psychic healer'. He soon picked up that I'd been sexually abused—I was so anxious. To help liberate me, he had me masturbate under a sheet while he went off and swung a crystal around. Then he came and fondled me himself.

'Okay,' I thought, 'therapists are OUT.' This kept me from my best source of help for another four years.

By this time I was 27. There was a kind older man whose sobriety group I attended. One day I burst into tears, and counselling soon began. I figured, 'He's older, he's married, and he's a long time sober—he's a safe bet.' For two years I worked on trusting him, on trying to accept that there really are good men, learning to discount my negative perceptions. He was the first person ever to validate my childhood sexual abuse. He kicked a chair over (great!) and said, 'The rotten bastard!' He was gentle and kind, and I cried on his shoulder once. We used to end the sessions with a hug.

After two years he made a pass at me. Instantly, I felt myself falling away, feeling 'I can only trust me'. He made another pass, and I was totally torn between the warmth and excitement, and repulsion. I went right into childlike feelings I didn't know I had—feeling that I was to blame, paranoid, and that 'no one must know—I'll kill myself first'. Afraid, split, confused.

I blamed my body. From that time, I had keen urges to self-mutilate. I wasn't going to try and recover again, and I dived into drink, tranquillisers, prostitution. One night I angrily slashed my legs, then put the razor to my wrist—but then thought, put it off just one more day. After six weeks, I got to detox in a very sick state. I had no idea how sick I was, till withdrawal began. It was hell on earth. I felt such pain and despair. In order to stay alive, I felt I had to trust someone. So I trusted the female psychologist, Jan; I talked of the abuse.

Then Jan calls me into her office. She says, 'You've talked to all these people. Whose response are you going to believe? Are you going to dine off this the rest of your life? Are you going to talk about it when you're admitted to a psychiatric hospital? I suggest you bury it.'

I returned to my bed in extreme pain, still withdrawing, and in no fit state to leave. She's wrong, she's right, she's wrong! I returned to Sydney drinking, and went for help again. I felt like such a hopeless case. I was 30.

After Jan, I avoided help for another four months, except for lots of AA. My state of mind was very bad, and I didn't feel I was worth helping. This nearly drove me back to the drink. I'd heard of Jim, another psychologist, and how kind he was. He is an expert on alcoholism. At seven months sober, I finally contacted him. I wasn't too keen on him being a man, that's for sure. The first time I attended Jim's group I was pleased—I could see that he was understanding, trustworthy and competent. But my ability to trust had been shattered. I thought, 'This is a laugh—at last I meet someone trustworthy, and now I can't do it!'

Jim talked to me after the group. I am an acute anxiety case.

He gently asks if I was abused as a child. 'Yes.' 'Sexually?' I am scared to say so, after the responses I'd had before. Maybe he'll say I'm 'dining off it' too. 'Yes, sexually.' He is very kind. Thank God!

Jim also asked what I thought I needed. 'I think I need a bit of support,' I reply. This was some understatement! He told me some time later that his first impression of me was of someone who was totally lost.

Today, nine years later, I'm happily nine years sober. I've been in the hospital where Jim works about 25 times, and attended masses of groups as an outpatient. I'm on medication, and have seen psychiatrists for seven years.

These difficulties stem from both the childhood abuse and my adult experiences when seeking help. Jim has proved highly trustworthy, though I still struggle on the trust front.

The bulk of the remembering happened a few years ago, which put me in hospital for 10 weeks. I trusted Jim like no other, and told him things I never thought I could tell a soul. He had all the time in the world for me then, and I just felt so loved and cared about. Lots of other people have helped—Rape Crisis have been wonderful—but I don't think I'd have remained sober or become as free of torment as I have, if it weren't for this one man's guidance. Jim has shown me that it is possible for a man to be fully loving, kind, patient. He's taught me a lot.

Wendy Nelson

◆

One thing I love about a good therapist is that when I'm bogged down in the mire of viewing a thing one way only, she offers all sorts of different perspectives while still allowing me to own my process.

I have worked very successfully (I measure this in terms of healing) with an amazing woman called Fran. She is reliable, genuinely values me, can hear the worst, validates me and is honest about her own limitations. What a gem!

Some years ago I visited a psychiatrist who told me how seductive little girls can be, and asked me terribly sexually intrusive questions. He suggested that I was getting off on the whodunnit aspect of my abuse memories; that if something had happened to me, so what, and that 'these social workers' encourage victims to 'wallow too much' in sexual assault. I got worse. With Fran, I've got better.

As your intuition develops, it becomes easier to tell whether a certain therapist is right for you or not.

Louise Plummer

◆

It's an ongoing process, this 'healing' business. There are stages, from being so utterly miserable that while you desperately want not to exist you have no energy at all to act on suicidal thoughts, to my present condition which is one of general happiness and hope. Even so, I am still on the journey to recovery: at any time, given a trigger—a sight, a smell, a sound—I am likely to experience irrational thoughts, rage or depression. Fortunately, such occurrences are rare these days.

During the most chaotic times of my breakdown, there were 'saviours'. One was a reformed drug addict and alcoholic, a friend of a friend, who spoke long-distance to me on the phone when I was in crisis. She would instruct me to simply breathe with her for five or ten minutes; sometimes she would send me off to undertake specific physical activities, such as vacuuming the loungeroom or folding the washing, before ringing her back. She advised me to play CDs of New Age music and to undertake a 12-step recovery programme. She told me the story of her own abuse, which was somewhat similar to mine, and tried to encourage me to believe that I would survive my sometimes overwhelming memories of being abused physically and sexually.

Two valuable ways of healing yourself, I believe, are to find an occupation you care about—whether it is income-producing or a hobby—and become immersed in it, and to try to help others. Both these are impossible when you are in chaos and barely able to function, but they do help to distance you from your own problems when you are able to function on a more even level.

My first two female therapists would sometimes physically hold me during therapy sessions. When they 'abandoned' me for the school holidays to be with their own children, I experienced intense feelings of grief and of wanting to harm myself. My pain at their withdrawal was an agonising echo of my mother's abandonment of me.

I had to wait seven long months before I was able to have regular sessions with my third, and current, therapist, a consultant psychiatrist. She set very firm boundaries with me during our initial sessions. These included no physical contact, and ample notification of forthcoming holiday breaks. Other factors that had caused problems with my first two therapists—such as my giving gifts, writing them letters trying to locate their homes—were not allowed, and strict conditions about after-hours contact also formed part of our written agreement.

My new therapist agreed not to talk about her personal life, and always to be on time beginning and ending our sessions (both my previous therapists were often late beginning sessions, which had added to my feelings of abandonment.)

In the 18 months I've been in therapy with my current doctor, my emotional health has improved greatly. I've been able to resume a normal professional and social life, something I had at one time believed would never be possible again. I haven't formed any real emotional bond with the therapist, but I am grateful to her for being reliable and consistent in not breaking any part of our contract.

Grace Power

◆

My therapist, a psychiatrist, has never once made leading suggestions about the cause of my breakdown, and the uncovering of memories has proceeded at my pace.

Jan Watson

✦

I was fortunate in finding people who were very gentle, caring and understanding. I worked with a number of different people over the years, including a man (often with his wife there or at least around) who, although he was not experienced in handling abuse cases, nevertheless did much to help me, including a brilliant session when he enabled me to switch for the first time from fear of my father to anger towards him. What stood out for me in each case was their willingness to listen, to be able to validate my feelings, to respect me as a person and where I was coming from, and to work with me acknowledging my own awareness of what I needed at the time. Having worked on a particular issue I appreciated being able to reflect, with the counsellor, on what had happened and to begin to integrate the memory I had recovered.

One of the most significant aspects for me was sensitive use of touch. To experience the deepest levels of pain I nearly always needed to be held, often with me gripping the other person. Sometimes just fingertip touch was enough to give me the confidence to keep going. One counsellor in particular had an amazing sensitivity to the need to remain silent for extended periods, and just to let me experience what was going on for me. Such times were generally very meaningful. The same counsellor effectively chooses from a wide range of methods available to her to access underlying pain.

Julie Waddy

Therapy that encourages embracing and valuing the child within is what I personally have found useful. Many people are currently pooh-poohing this as New Age nonsense, but it has worked for me. It makes perfect sense to me to give that little one now what she did not have then. How beautiful it is that it isn't too late— this has been the triumph and central tenet of my healing.

A very skilled and supportive therapist is needed here, as some of those regressive, pain-filled times can be truly frightening. I remember doing a John Bradshaw meditation some time ago. It was very powerful and ultimately positive, but I'd unfortunately disregarded his caution about grounding oneself and having a support person on standby. This really is necessary; without it, I walked around carrying the horrible, knee-buckling grief of my five-year-old self for about a week. I knew it was this little girl's buried pain I was releasing, but I also had to carry her other feelings, such as black, suicidal self-hatred. If you are doing this sort of painful but transforming work, *do not do it alone*.

Working with your younger selves is like healing from the foundations up, and today a sense of love and innocence I never thought possible fills me when I look at Little Louise. I'm also very good mates with my inner 14-year-old. The difficulty is in moving through the hatred of self put into those kids. However, it is possible.

Here is a poem I wrote for my four-year-old self that might illustrate the beauty of the change that can take place.

TO MY INFANT RECLAIMED
I called you from the shadowed path
And told you, 'I am thine'.
I saw your little tearstained face
And said, 'Come, you are mine'.
I spread my arms and beckoned
As I yearned for your sweet embrace.
I whispered, 'Little one,
I've come to take you from this place'.
At first you were reluctant

After years of scorn and hate,
But then you ran right up to me
And said, 'It's not too late'.
With wildest joy I scooped you up
Your tears blending with my own
For I am you and you are me
Tho' twenty years have flown.
I wrenched you from Svengali's grasp
And said, 'Take my hand, let's go'.
I washed your wounds and held you
Never more to let you go.
And when I looked to see you
You'd gone inside of me,
Washed of shame and innocent
Now, child, we are set free

Louise Plummer

◆

From psychiatry to some alternative methods, I've experienced many forms of therapy. As a man working his way through the maze of therapies available I would say that they all contributed something, though some were more helpful than others. Bearing in mind that men tend to have difficulty experiencing and expressing our feelings, I found the 'experiential' therapies the most beneficial, though they were difficult. The 'talk' therapies were easy and comfortable, which is often what's not needed to effect change and release. They're great at the beginning of therapy to get people used to talking about themselves, and again at the end when explanation is helpful.

It's especially difficult for we men to reveal all to a therapist or group, particularly for the first time. A good therapist is aware of this. I would especially look out for acknowledgement as a significant indicator of a good therapist. Next would come challenge or gentle push; challenge and encouragement to express the real feelings around the abuse will also help you to understand and to think helpfully about your experiences.

I would steer well clear of interpretive, emotionally restrained, judgemental, interventionist and airy-fairy therapists. I would be extremely suspicious of—and would actually walk out on—any therapist who proclaims his/her approach to be the best, or who runs down other approaches. I have experienced this with some older (particularly male) psychiatrists.

Taylor Shane

✦

I have worked with two therapists—the first was wonderful and the second woeful. The first was a very caring, wise and under-standing psychologist. We worked together for five years. He never tried to control my behaviour, and never demanded I do anything against my will. He'd always listen and accept my feelings and methods of dealing with issues. He taught and encouraged me to hear my inner child, my gut, my body and my heart's feelings. He'd often give me cuddles, which helped me to move through my intense pain and reconnect to the normal need for loving touch. Overall he helped me to save my mental and emotional health from completely crumbling because of the horrendous effects of my childhood abuse and neglect. He is a model therapist and a man I'll be always be grateful to.

For three months I worked with a female therapist who had no training. Her honesty, initial kind words, admiration for me and her caring touch (she's a masseuse) kept me from leaving her, though the wise part of me kept saying she wasn't suitable. I was desperate for loving attention, and felt I'd take whatever support she could provide. I feel bad about this now. I wish I'd listened to my wise voice, but I know I did my best. She believed I'd heal only if I allowed myself to be her puppet, that is, to let her take over. But after three months she decided that she was out of her depth and without notice told me she was ending our therapy. I was shocked, found it hard to talk, felt rejected and overwhelmed. As I sat in front of her in this state she repeatedly told me that she didn't like the way I was behaving, that she wanted us to talk like adults and I was being stupid and childish. To top it off she asked me to call her and thank her for ending our therapeutic relationship as she was doing it for my benefit. I walked away in tears feeling very alone. That was the last time I saw her.

Still grieving over the loss of my first therapist I now had to deal with another loss. After talking about it with friends I decided to write and let her know that her behaviour was unprofessional and unacceptable. Initially I had felt I was to blame—that is, my being a survivor of sexual and satanic ritual abuse made it unbearable for her to be around me. Generally I feel this way with a lot of people. I now know that this wasn't the cause of her unprofessional behaviour or the reason she ended therapy. My lesson from this has been always to listen to my wise voice, even if it means leaving someone when I am feeling desperate for caring attention. I am working hard at reparenting myself, and I am healing. My advice to other survivors is to work only with a qualified therapist who does not try to control your behaviour, who respects and believes you at all times, and who encourages you to love yourself.

Skyy Bright

◆

THE HEALING PROCESS

Are there any clues that healing is taking place? Survivors' stories attest to the fact that there definitely are signs: the feeling of being overwhelmed by it all, the terror and disorientation, begin to lessen; you will have good moments, good hours, good days. You will see glimpses of hope in the moments when you succeed in doing something that once would have been beyond you—the smallest step is still a step forward.

Patience is a difficult virtue for a survivor, though the child part of ourselves has often been practising it for many years, waiting for the time to be right to tell her or his story. There is so much pain that often all you want is to be rid of it—not to feel that you are going mad, to be able to stop clenching your jaw to the point of tears, to be able to stand in the light and not hide, to feel safe and unafraid, to feel 'good' instead of 'bad', to be able to make your own choices in your own best interests rather than feeling like a puppet whose strings are being pulled by your past. But you cannot simply get rid of the pain: you have to feel it fully in order to be released from it. If you try to deny it or fight it, you are fighting yourself. Stay with it, honour it, honour yourself for surviving at all. The journey takes patience as well as courage.

The precise steps in the healing journey are different for each survivor. Nevertheless, there are common themes running through all these accounts, particularly a sense of coming home and of discovering the power of love—for others and for ourselves. It is love that abuse betrays; it is love that healing restores.

WHEN A CHILD CRIES
A child cries—
and a little brat fights back.
A child yearns for love—
It's received with a thump and a slap.
A child wants freedom—to run, be alive—
this is fulfilled with crap, hurt and lies.
A child wants to be safe and secure—
this is provided with a sexual lure.
A child wants to be held, and told it's all right—
not always abused and told to be quiet.
A child wants to have a place to belong—
not told to get lost and always to be wrong.
A child suffers pain much more than adults—
then suffers the grief and believes it's their fault.
A child has the strength to cope and endure
beyond all pain, beyond all lures.

A child lies huddled, curled up in its room
with a cloud of darkness, and one of doom.
A child takes its last breath, then disappears—
with it she takes her sadness and tears.
A child lies huddled in an old lifeless shell—
To symbolise the torture and all of the hell.
Goodbye my child, for now you are free—
I'll take your place, no more pain
will there be.

Karen J. Berthold

◆

One of the most fundamental tenets of my healing is that what is important is not so much what happened to me as the sense I have made of it. How wonderful this has been. I cannot change what happened to me, but I can change the destructive messages it gave me about myself.

It began with my beginning to question what my abusers' words or deeds meant to me. Just because that was their view, does it have to be mine? I have adopted and integrated my own view of myself as worthy. Initially this was a very intellectual process: I had all the right words in my head, but still felt basically rotten inside. With time and love, I have accepted in all of me that I am not the disgusting things that were done to me.

I felt that my abusers had destroyed my dignity forever, and that I would never be able to live with what they did to me. Not true! It is my growing sense of worth that enables me to see the beauties that their lies hid from view.

Much of my healing has come from listening to others. There have been times when one short sentence has revolutionised me.

To my delight and surprise, I have also found many answers within me.

An important step in my healing was for me to let go of the need to know why it happened. I can't answer all of that; it is sufficient for my 'inner child' and I to know why it didn't: it didn't happen because I was bad or deserved it. I understand what it wasn't about, and that is enough.

Moving on is wonderful. I remember getting my first 'A' for an essay at university. I drove home crying and feeling really confused. I was supposed to be stupid and unable to do anything right ... wasn't I? By whose definition? The abusers'! It's not mine any longer.

Now that I am where I am, I feel such hurt and anger for some of the beautiful survivors I know who cannot see their gifts. Not yet, anyway. I continue to support and affirm their worth, and believe that they will come to know what I do: that the grief for a stolen childhood is really powerful. I thought I would never stop crying once I reached this stage. I did, though. Rage expressed at the right people is also essential to healing. How dare anyone so devalue a child?

If abuse damage spreads into all areas of a person, so too does the magic of healing.

For people with recovered memories who may, as I did, despair of ever coming to terms with their abuse, I'd like to say, you will. My experience of this stage was possibly the hardest, as the grief was so enormous. I could understand very well why I hadn't wanted to believe these things; not only are they horrific and scary, but they are so very, very sad. At one stage I could not even refer to my abuse in passing without being consumed by terrible pain, but this was born of a growing love for that little girl within me.

I came through. Hang in there: you will too. Do not be deterred. There are wonderful parts of you that your abuser/s did not reach.

Louise Plummer

◆

Healing from abuse is a spiral process in my experience. I find that when I think I have finally learned that piece of behaviour or healed that part of my life for good, inevitably it arises again in a slightly different guise somewhere along the line, showing me that the damage has been multifaceted. It has touched most if not all aspects of my life. It is hard. It is lonely. It is painful. At times it is even very scary, and drives you to regard death as a peaceful release from the constant struggle.

It gets better. It eases. Most of all what I like is that it shows me how interesting a person I am. I am unique. There is no one else exactly like me on this planet. What gets me through is my sense of humour and my great imagination!

What I found more than anything else in my healing journey is—it takes courage, and you have to do it yourself.

Peter Sandford

◆

People have often tried to tell me this and tell me that, what I should and shouldn't do, and a whole lot of other things— much of this I call abuse. For me, healing from my wounds has come as a product of my own efforts, increased understanding, and the love, empathy and understanding that others have shown me.

I often tried to emphasise to my previous therapists that my problems were quite normal and understandable if they could see me as a human being who had been wounded and who needed some support to get back on my feet, and if they saw themselves as human beings too—instead of having these funny scientific concepts of what a human being is supposed to be, categorising 'normal' and 'abnormal' thoughts, feelings, behaviours, and thinking about how they could 'fix' my problems.

For me healing is about recognising all the injustices, becoming sensitive to and aware of all the suffering and pain that people go through and try and numb themselves to. Healing is about reclaiming my power, my balance, my awareness, my wildness, my sensitivity, my place in nature, in the universe—I'm not here to be 'normal' or 'healthy'. It has helped me to lift up my voice and speak, to tell, to let my voice be heard.

John Tardy

✦

My grandfather began abusing me when I was only three years old. Much later in my adult life, when my grandmother died I began to experience difficulties in many areas. I began to do things that were out of character for me, and I constantly felt angry. I experienced difficulties in so many areas of my life that I finally decided to consult my parish priest. The unconditional love that he showed me got me on the way to healing, but there was still a great deal of work to do.

I did two things that helped me: I found a therapist, and I completed a course for victims of abuse. The crucial factor in my healing was deciding that I wanted to live. I needed not to be stuck in myself. Also, my husband became ill and I had a new baby. I nursed my husband and my baby and I learned new ways to nurture myself.

Now I can eat a cake or chocolates if I want them. I take myself for a massage, which is something I never would have done for myself in the past. I sometimes put myself before the children and take myself off for the day. It's OK to go away and spend time on myself. I got back the power to say NO.

Family counselling was very helpful—we all had the opportunity to talk about our feelings. The ability to speak was as important for the rest of the family as it was for me. For so long I had taken my anger out on them.

Now I know who I can trust, I have instincts. Not to feel bad about trusting someone is wonderful. I have the new skill of being honest—a wonderful gift I will never lose again.

I can't talk about my healing without speaking of my faith. I have a deep and abiding faith in God and I know that I was brought to this point in my life for a reason. It's all in God's divine plan. I know that good will always come from bad if we just allow it.

I have a saying in my mind, 'My grandfather stole my colour'. For most of my life I have not been able to distinguish the beautiful and exquisite colours, smells, feelings and sensations that other people have always spoken about. They were just not there for me. Some time after my healing was well on its way I travelled on a train across from Western Australia back to Sydney. I looked out of the window and suddenly—there it was, Dorothea Mackellar's beautiful sunburnt country! I had never had the ability to see such beauty before, and now I could. I sat on that train and cried all the way to Sydney. Now my garden is always full of roses. For me the roses represent the beauty, colour and sensation that my grandfather stole. They also represent the eternal hope of a new spring blossoming, of healing and redemption.

Elizabeth McMinn

✦

My sister and I were sexually abused by our father. I believe he had intercourse with my sister when she was 12, and I was touched by him penetrating me with his finger when I was six. He did this whenever my mother was out at meetings at night, I believe for a couple of years.

There was an awkward silence—and still is—about what happened. I believe others in my family are in denial, or don't want to face the reality. It was all reported to the police but he was never charged.

I am now 22 years old and I feel optimistic and excited about the future. I have a supportive boyfriend and I feel I am finding my place in the world, going to university and also coming to terms with what happened.

A positive legacy from my father is that I have a good brain and I intend to use it in pursuit of justice. I want answers to questions such as what motivates people to commit these acts despite their natural sense of right and wrong. I would like my father to realise the effect his abuse had on me. I only had love and admiration for him and I find it hard to understand how he could betray that so selfishly. I know that somewhere inside my father is the real victim, because there is a part of himself that he hides from—and that is a lifelong jail sentence.

I make an effort not to dwell on the past. I want to resolve this in a healthy, positive way and have a life.

Alison McDougal

I decided that I would need a place to go, a sanctuary, where I could go within, a place where I would be safe to think, to cry, to heal. My husband suggested that I use the back room. He invited me to set it up just as I would like. It was to be my little room.

The child within me loved that room. My friends called it the 'spirit-filled room'—their title was apt. I came to know my child in this place. She was safe here, safe to express all she felt.

Jacinta McMurray

My healing began when I was involved in a self-help course called 'Money and You'. Due to the intense emotional growth exercises employed during the course, I had what can be termed a 'spontaneous rebirth'. I got in touch with parts of my psyche I had buried and forgotten. This led me to seek more experiences in this area. I participated in rebirthing classes, and finally undertook a course to become a rebirther myself. I also took part in reiki and other bodywork courses. I found that I had the ability to access 'the moment of pure bliss'—a moment so wonderful that it has kept me pursuing my journey. My involvement with the men's movement has healed my mistrust of my own manhood.

During my search, I discovered that I am personally responsible for my own responses. What was done to me is now no longer relevant. I am responsible. I can change the tapes that play in my inner thoughts all day and all night. I am able, if I wish, to open up and accept pure love. I have accessed my own power. I have undergone many processes to clear self-sabotaging thoughts.

My self-esteem varies from day to day, but generally it is high. The thought I would like to leave with you is this, quoted by a teacher of mine: If you always do what you've always done, you'll always get what you've always got.

Phillip Harrison

◆

After a period of dealing with a therapist, I found that I was still feeling depressed and sad. I felt it was time for me to get out of the rut I was in. It seemed to me that I spent far too much time on myself and dwelling on my own problems. The therapist helped me to work through them, but after that it was up to me to do something about my own life.

I decided to do the telephone volunteer's course with the Sydney City Mission. One night during the course we were asked to draw a picture of our childhood home, to draw all our family members in their rightful places in the house, and then to put ourselves in the house. I found that I couldn't do it—I could not go back into that house!

When we were asked to describe our drawings, I couldn't bring myself to talk about mine and was excused from the exercise. Later I realised that I never, ever had to go into that house again.

A huge support to me during my healing was the time I spent volunteering on the mission telephones. The feeling that I could do something to help others was tremendously restorative. There are so many people with terribly sad lives, reaching out for help from just about any direction. It made me see that I was much farther along in my healing than I had previously thought. That was the beginning of getting well for me, of healing from my abuse.

May Smith

◆

When I was a teenager living in a home where I felt afraid, scrutinised and oppressed, one of my outlets was music. To sit down in the loungeroom and play the piano and sing songs was an escape from my fearful reality. I didn't even consciously think about myself as finding a way out or a way through the pain of emotional abuse. Yet there was a blissful hiding place in the notes of the music that filled the air and filled my heart.

I've been writing music for half my life, and playing the piano since I was six years old—more than 20 years. It's something that has always been there in my life, and I couldn't imagine life without it.

Abuse is something that's always been there too. The sexual abuse lasted nine years, and in my teenage years the emotional abuse followed. My life was always shaped by the fear of the seemingly all-powerful one—my father.

And my father is tone deaf! A coincidence, perhaps? Music always created a world for me that no one else could enter, and of course my father was not welcome, with his monotone voice and his impatience with complex rhythms. He would say to me, 'That sounds great—to a deaf person!' His spiteful humour only served to encourage me to do what he scoffed at.

As the years have gone by, music has become less of an escape and more of an expression. For me, healing and music go hand in hand. As I have written songs that express my pain and my questioning of the suffering in the world and in my life, I have found an outlet for the pain. This eventually resulted in the production of two albums of my songs. The first was about the role of a good

God in the context of suffering; the second is an expression of the issues that arose in my adult life in the wake of abuse as a child.

After the release of *Only The Suffering God* I received letters from all over the country thanking me, but people sometimes seemed a bit puzzled that I could write music which grapples with complex questions without providing any answers. I have come to realise that answers don't come easily, and what really helps others who are suffering is an identification with the problem, not a glib answer.

When the second album, *The Lies of Love*, is released, it will expose me as a survivor of abuse to anyone who cares to listen to the music. That frightens me in part, but also makes me proud— proud of the healing work I have done, and proud that I no longer feel too ashamed of my past to let people know that I have survived.

Mono

◆

My healing began during my thirties. At that time I undertook a rebirthing class. During the rebirthing I came in contact with my own terror and my body memories. After that experience I started to deal slowly with the memories and the feelings they produced in me. I became deathly ill, and no doctor could find a physiological cause. I knew that I was a bad person and felt that if anything or anyone ever hurt me, it must inevitably be my fault.

After my marriage to my present husband I began to work at my healing the only way that I know how—110 per cent. There are some days even now when the feelings are raw and I have terrible fear, but they are rare. Also I am married to a wonderful man who knows instantly what is happening to me. He reassures me that I am here and I am safe, which helps me tremendously. I tried conventional therapy, but for me it was not as successful as the rebirthing. I find that my mind cannot stand being still for very long; meditation makes me feel uncomfortable.

I still have a problem with self-esteem. It is a great effort to maintain the front, the apparent confidence that everyone sees in me. I still feel angry that the abuse happened to me and that no charges were ever laid. The experience has caused me to feel pathological fear, to the point of not being able to breathe if I don't know where my daughters are every second of the day and night.

But I am here, and I am safe, and so is my family. That is enough for now.

Elizabeth Quinn

◆

There is a lot of hard, tedious work I have to do to overcome the ingrained, distorted, yucky beliefs about myself. Simple things like putting on a jumper when I'm cold. How do I know I am cold, when I am not in my body? I have had to learn to be in my body and literally to 'come to my senses'.

Coming to my senses. A scary idea, when my senses have been constantly assaulted. So I started to please my senses, to encourage them to function again.

Touch: Gently touch my skin. Feels nice. Buy a silk shirt. Feels wonderful. Stroke my cat. Soft fur.

Smell: Potpourri on my bedside table. What a lovely smell! Lavender bags in my wardrobe. A dab of sandalwood on my wrist, so I can occasionally sniff it throughout the day.

Hearing: Birds in the morning. Take a minute to listen to their song. Classical music. Quiet and pleasing to my ears. My lover telling me how gorgeous I am. Yes, I'll listen to that!

Taste: Leatherwood honey from Tasmania. Tangy and sweet. Earl Grey tea. Tingles my tongue. Biting into a watermelon. Yum!

Seeing: Fresh flowers on my kitchen table. Nice poster on the wall. Flying pig hanging from the ceiling. What a great place to come home to!

Coming back to my senses, returning to my body, also means that I will stop self-abusive behaviour, that I get a quality mattress so I can have a good night's sleep, that I have my teeth checked regularly. Oh, how very scary for a ritual abuse survivor! But if I visit the dentist every six months, there is never much to repair.

It also means learning how to breathe again. Have you noticed how often we hold our breath? Take a deep breath right now!

It also means taking exercise: to walk, swim, cycle or better still, to learn self-defence, which not only keeps me fit but also teaches me that yes, there is a way out—and that I am worth defending.

Returning to my body, coming to my senses, also brought the most difficult task of all—to feel! Unfortunately, learning to feel also means feeling the bad feelings and the pain. But in the meantime I have learned that feeling even the bad feelings will eventually result in my feeling good. Feeling good happens more and more often these days.

Phoenix Van Dyke

◆

My main source of strength came from setting the goal to finish my counselling course and become a counsellor so that I could leave my job as a teacher and begin the work that I really wanted to do. I would be able to walk out of a situation which was unhealthy for me and in which I felt trapped.

I am much better now than I have been in a long time. I am still healing. I am in a nurturing relationship with a person who is wonderful. I am beginning to be able to trust, not only other people but my own feelings. I learned a great deal about boundaries from a book about codependence. I now know that I have needs, and I have learnt to ask the little girl inside me what it is she needs. I listen to her, and I give her what she needs. As the fourth child in my family, I always felt the responsibility of looking after everyone else's emotional needs. Now I try to look after mine. When things were really bad, I allowed myself to ring the helplines.

I light candles for myself and look at them to centre myself. I have flowers around me. Sometimes I go to bed, even if it's four o'clock in the afternoon, if that is what I need to do for myself. I can now say on a bad day, 'Tomorrow is another day'.

My message is that there is always a huge hope for healing. In order to nurture our own healing, we need to be around people who believe in us and who support us. We need to share in the strength of others and not allow ourselves to be alone.

Healing has taken place for me because of:
• a fantastic therapist
• healing tools, e.g. left-hand writing and drawing
• reading books on healing, e.g. *The Courage to Heal*
• changing my work and being around supportive people
• telling my story in a group
• new 'self-talk', e.g. telling myself I am safe, I am an adult now, I have choices
• doing nurturing things, e.g. making a hot bowl of soup or having a rest
• doing my 'family of origin' work
• being in a new relationship with someone who is also healing, and is very aware.

Elizabeth Jane Frost

✦

My past experience of being 'crazy' is a painful thing to write about, but I feel I've reached the stage of being able to be more open about it. Many people suffer from various forms of psychosis. I healed from it naturally—that is, without medication—while in intensive psychotherapy, and I strongly believe others can do the same. I now see my 'craziness' more as the after-effects of the extreme abuse I was forced to endure by my sadistic-psychopathic uncle and his vile friends. Blocking out the abuse kept me alive, but later I paid a heavy price in emotional and mental health.

I felt that my mind was being squeezed, as though someone's

hand was inside my head, holding my brain and squeezing it. This was mental torture. I could feel a constant pain in my chest, terror, shame, guilt, self-hate, agony . . . I kept asking myself why, but I had no answers. I just felt the need to keep running, to hide from the world. I felt I was to be killed, or that I'd drop dead from a fatal disease. I could feel my blood clotting, sometimes every day. My head was always in a foggy state, everything inside my body and around me terrified me. Everything I heard—television, radio, people talking—would go around in my head until I thought my brain would explode. I'd find lumps I believed were cancer.

My parents were distressed about my condition but didn't know what to do. They just wanted me to get better, get my act together. My therapist, who I began to see two years after I first began to experience the mental torture, was the only person who completely understood and cared. I couldn't have made it without his support.

Once I began to remember about my horrific childhood the 'craziness' occurred less often. The more I remembered and connected with my inner child, the less crazy I became. I had suffered horrendous physical, mental and emotional pain, and nearly died several times. That is why my mind had been so tortured with the fear of dying. My intense fears were all related to real incidents from the dreadful sexual and satanic ritual abuse I had endured as a child.

I believe that all our thoughts are linked to our experiences, that there is a reason for everything; I believe that insanity is seldom a chemical disorder. More often, it is the mind trying to tell us of issues we need to face. Once we face them and reconnect with our beautiful inner child in loving ways, we begin to heal. I still have a lot of fears, and am continuing to work intensely on my healing—the amount of extreme abuse I suffered was very great. I'm glad to say that I haven't been 'crazy' for years. I don't need to be any more, as I've remembered what I needed to know.

There's a quote I used to read a lot to help me get through the times I felt 'crazy' and suicidal. It's from a book called *Healing*

Your Aloneness by Dr E. Chopich and Dr M. Paul. I think the authors are harsh to call us self-abusers for acting out towards ourselves what was done to us as children, but I agree with their theories. Here's the quote:

'The deepest pain that we have to face is the aloneness and lone-liness and the wrenching experience of powerlessness with respect to those feelings that we experienced as children. *All our craziness is caused by our reluctance to experience these feelings.* All our ego protections start with the fear of that pain.

The severity of mental illness from which a person suffers is directly related to the degree of internal disconnection between Inner Adult and Inner Child. *Craziness results when we avoid feeling and facing the deep aloneness and pain of the Inner Child.'*

I'm aware that many people would disagree with this, and see mental illness as something medication can fix. I think that med-ication is a short-term fix, and for full recovery to take place healing between the Inner Adult and Inner Child is needed. It worked for me, and I'm sure it can work for others. I'm not saying that no one should take medication, but it alone won't heal our minds, hearts and souls.

Skyy Bright

◆

After 12 years of sobriety from all drugs and alcohol I've decided to take anti-depressant medication—Prozac. This decision has left me feeling like a terrible failure and full of shame at times. The decision took me months of consideration and turmoil, but now after three months of taking it I am able to talk more openly about it.

I have chronic post-traumatic stress disorder (PTSD). One of the challenges I face is 'Affect Tolerance and Affect Modulation'—a comforting medical term for handling my overwhelming feelings.

I have learned to regulate my emotions by using a visualisation of a small control panel with four knobs of different colours representing a certain feeling: red for anger, green for anxiety, blue for sadness, black for fear/depression. I can often effectively lower anxiety, fear, sadness, depression and anger levels just by visualising the control knobs and turning down the 'volume' of that emotion. With practice I have become quite adept at this.

However, there was a period when the urge to end it all was frequently overwhelming me, and I became frightened of what I might do. I was almost constantly focused on modulating my depression control knob and turning it down. It was exhausting, and took most of my concentration. Eventually I gave in, and succumbed to the 'medication cop-out'!

I now wonder what took me so long. Why was I so slow in taking this extremely helpful medication? It has saved my life, and has given me the stability to explore some of the more scary parts of my childhood. It's as though the part of my unconscious that has been protecting me all my life (particularly through blocking any memory of the abuse) wasn't allowing some of the worst of it to surface while there was a chance of my suiciding as a result of reliving those experiences.

I do know why it took me so long. Everywhere in my group, medication is slandered. It is seen as a cop-out, a means of numbing the pain and of avoidance. This makes me angry, as it prevented me from utilising a fantastic resource earlier, and I worry about the many survivors who never try this route. As a drug and alcohol counsellor I am constantly faced with the problems that over-prescribing or inappropriate use of prescription drugs can cause in people's lives. The anti-medication forum has grown out of this huge problem, and understandably so. But we have the right to choose; part of reclaiming our power is to have options and to discern what is right for us.

Recent research shows that those of us with PTSD often have an imbalance in the neurochemicals in our brains. Serotonin is one of these, and fluoxetine hydrochloride (Prozac) is an effective means of stabilising it. What a relief! I don't see myself taking it forever, only while I am processing the worst of my memories. This may free me at last from 30 years of suffering.

Ineke Veerkamp

◆

There have been many stages in my healing process.
- The first thing I had to face in coming to terms with my sexual abuse was the shock, horror and total disbelief, as the pressure to remain silent can be very strong, and it really took a lot of work not to fall into the pattern of denial. I have found that directing my anger to help create change, and speaking out, have been very healing. It is vitally important to speak out so others know that they are not alone, and that healing is possible no matter what they have been through.
- The crisis point was when I would age-regress to the child and relive the trauma. I learned to remind myself that it wasn't happening now, and found that by feeling the pain and not fighting it, I felt better.
- I would go from not being able to speak about it to wanting to tell the world. Group work was my greatest healing tool, as I met other survivors who were willing to work on themselves, and speaking about it has been so healing, especially when others can relate to what you are going through. This has been a source of strength and encouragement.
- The feelings of powerlessness and being vulnerable immobilised me. All I could do was stay in bed and rest. Fortunately I had loving support from my husband, who took care of me when I was at my worst.
- Body memories, flashbacks and nightmares were the worst, though I noticed after doing a reiki course of natural healing that they disappeared.
- Anger and hatred have been very strong emotions to work

through. I don't believe that you can just 'think' forgiveness and be completely healed. The hurt suffered needs to be healed before forgiveness can take place. I am replacing the anger and hatred with love; this has been a gradual, freeing process for me.

- Hurting the self is something I no longer need to do, as I have learned to make it okay to feel and release my emotions. Since I have had counselling and done group work I have been able to integrate and feel like a real person. I am in the process of becoming whole and healed. Recovery is worth the effort.
- Lack of trust is another big area to deal with. I found that the healthier I became by working through my pain, the more I was able to learn to trust my intuition. I no longer take to heart put-downs from insensitive or hurtful people.
- In the past, I had difficulty nurturing and taking care of myself. I am now getting adequate sleep, exercise, healthy food and not pushing myself too hard. Massage, hot baths, reading, writing and speaking are helping me tap into my creativity, which has been vital to my healing.
- The biggest difficulty for me has been my damaged self-esteem, and I am pleased to say that today I am doing things I never thought possible. It took a lot to work through the negativity and pain, but it was worth it. Because I was always putting myself down I had to learn to recognise and acknowledge all the progress and steps I made along the way, and I kept a record of these.
- The greatest challenge was to learn to love myself, and not to carry the shame or blame that we have all been led to believe is true. The sad fact was that everything I had been told made me feel so flawed and defective. This hindered my life and blocked me from success, but at 37 I feel now I am truly learning to live, and I see the world through the eyes of a child as a magical and mystical place.

• The thing I have found to be my greatest strength, even though I have had to face my dark nights of the soul in my recovery, is my spiritual belief. I know that in my call for help, I have been assisted in coming so far.

Linda Honey

✦

Until recently I hated parts of me being touched, and most men could not understand this so would try to force me to accept their advances. Now I have dealt with the abuse in my childhood I understand that the teacher (my abuser) focused on these parts of me. Since being in therapy I no longer have this problem. I lost 23 years of my life trying to self-destruct, never understanding why. Finally my life has meaning.

Kym Dunbar

✦

Many times I have felt there was only death in living and that I would die from the overwhelming sadness I have experienced. Although I am still healing from all of this, I have some of the happiness of the rainbow after the rain, as one friend said. I still take heed of the voice inside of me that says, 'You will make it' and 'Do not give up'. I consider myself on the way to being joyously free of a hideous past.

Penny Stevens

✦

I am a 54-year-old Sydney resident who grew up in middle-class comfort in an ambitious family environment. As an adult I was plagued with feelings of inadequacy, and struggled to be a super-person, to be all things to all people. It came a shock to me when I could no longer function in day-to-day life.

Five and a half years later I'm content, carefree, losing excess weight, free from the pain of muscle tension, and know that life *is* worthwhile. I won't lie and say it was easy—that wouldn't be fair to all survivors on the same journey. I will say that all the pain of recovering buried memories, along with the feelings of shame, blame and humiliation, are a necessary part of the healing process. In the end it's all worth it. Each of us alone knows our own pain as no one else can, and each of us alone deals with it the best way we can.

If I can do it, you can too. I'm not more clever, more lucky, more 'anything' than you. We all have the capacity to overcome the horrors of our childhood. It takes time, but the freedom from fear and from secrets is exhilarating. Trust yourself, reach out for help, and learn to trust others again.

Lyn

◆

I grew up not trusting anyone. Until 15 years ago I led a solitary existence. Now life is *so* much better. Therapy finished 18 months ago, and I am at peace with myself and the world. I am alive in a new way. During the 11 years of therapy, I required regular Valium and lived on chocolate. I have required neither since I finished therapy.

June Harcourt

◆

As I began my journey into recovery from ritual abuse, I had no idea where it would lead me, or that I could possibly know the hope and beauty of life as I know it today. It has not been easy and it still is not, but the path is lighter now and the future brighter.

When I entered recovery (or as I now refer to it, transformation or transcendence), I forgot the good stuff I had learned, which had enabled me to get through the 'shit'. I identified the past as all bad, discounting it. I left my survival skills behind, and then wondered why this healing was so tough to get through.

Instead of powering onward I became disempowered, helpless, a victim.

It was not until my counsellor challenged me to see that I was not progressing because I had stalled in the role of victim that I got in touch again with my inner strength. I took up the challenge, with a greater courage than ever before. I began to practise small safe steps, and little by little the risks I took to change began to transform me. This sounds easy; it was in fact excruciating and fear-laden, and I did many U-turns.

Life to me is a gift and a challenge. I am worthy of survival and more. 'Beyond the torment is a better way of living, and I will find it,' I said to myself. Underlying all the skills and support I got from my counsellor and friends was a drive to find meaning in all this. We know there is more to this world than what people can see. Ritual abuse survivors like us have seen the unseeable, the spiritual evil. I figured out that the love and goodness they hate so much must be the one thing they fear. I therefore went on a journey with the aim of finding love and goodness.

Along the way, people were kind to me. But I wanted more, I wanted to be loved for being a person in my own right, to stand proud! When times got tough I refused to give in. Stubbornly I kept motivated to know love in my life, as I know I was meant to do. There was no way I was going to die before I experienced its fullness.

The fact is that their threats failed. My father shot himself, my mother died diseased. The rest of them know they have lost, they could not contain me. Yee haa!

The monumental celebration to our existence is that we are here! We made it this far, we have what it takes to be more than an existence; to conquer and come home to love. I would imagine myself a mighty warrior, whom nothing could conquer. I had goodness and love, power and courage standing with me. I clothed myself in love, and the bonds of friendships were gilded in love's golden glow. How could I not win? I smile now, knowing the power of such imaginings. We can do anything.

Anna Foster

✦

Love. It's everything. We need to be loved, but even more we need to be able to love someone else. My parents denied me that, but I'm stubborn. I insist on loving. I insist on my own honesty. I hug my family and my friends. Some of them had trouble with that at first, but they're okay now. I've learned not to be intrusive; I've learned that I'm expected to have boundaries, and I need to respect other people's boundaries.

In healing I've learned that we're all different. We are all at different stages of growth, and that's okay. I've learned not to impose my standards, ideas, boundaries, limits, etc. on others. I love people. When a friend or relative does me a kindness I can tell them I appreciate it. I value their friendship. I look on my sisters as my friends, and vice versa.

My relationships are like a wheel. I am in the centre, my family and friends are around me in any position that they choose—as close or as distant as they wish to be. It's amazing that when I stopped trying to cling to my friends and gave them space, they came closer.

I am amazingly lucky with my friends. They actually like me for who I am, and not for who I thought they wanted me to be. I only have to be me—and they will like me anyway. I'm okay as I am.

Linley Valente

✦

My abuser told me I was bad and that I deserved to be punished. He told me in so many ways. By the words he said to me, by the way he treated me, and by the utter contempt in his eyes. Those eyes, so full of his own misery, reflected onto me. I have been living his version of me all of my life. What a waste.

My stepfather was abusive towards me sexually from the time I was eight years old. My mother, for reasons of her own, was a non-protecting parent. Fortunately or unfortunately, I managed to repress much of what happened to me until, in November 1994, at age 47 and after a traumatic accident, I began to remember. When the memories began to surface it was like being bludgeoned with a huge sledgehammer while standing in a wind tunnel with every ounce of air being sucked out of my lungs. I spent every waking moment feeling as though I would either die of suffocation or perish from the extreme pain and fear of it all. There are no words, really, to describe the pain.

I asked myself about a million times a day if I could be crazy. I asked my therapist about two million times if I could be crazy. My mother had suffered mental health problems, and I was terrified that I was beginning to follow in her footsteps. The flashbacks, body memories, anxiety attacks, the nightmares, the bed wetting, anorexia and the paralysing fear all told me that there was more to this than the delusions of a crazy person. Something real was happening to me that made me feel crazy.

My belief in my God has had a lot to do with my healing. I believe that God is love. I believe that love and time can heal anything. There have been so many times when I didn't think that I would ever get to the end of the pain. Gradually, little by little I began to feel parts of me shifting to something more peaceful, less tortured.

During the worst of it my kind and loving husband was there to support me. He witnessed the ugliness and the badness in me. He saw the terrible pain I was feeling and gently supported me, sometimes holding me while I cried, other times proclaiming his love for me, and sometimes just telling me again how brave and courageous he thought I was for facing the pain and fear and not running away. He did all the things for me that for a time I was unable to do for myself: he loved me, had faith in me, respected and admired me.

My therapist suggested that the little girl might be angry and need to express that rage. I waited until my family were all out of the house, then I put on my workout clothes and went to my son's bedroom. He has a punching bag, and I began to punch that bag and scream. It was the voice of the little girl, screaming at her stepfather. I punched until my arms were too tired to rise up any more, and then I cried. I was never allowed to cry when I was growing up. My stepfather told me that if I cried while he was hurting me he would kill my mother and then he would kill me, so I kept quiet.

Now I can scream, and I do. I cry and I yell and I scream, and he can never stop me again.

There were many times when I sat in my therapist's office and cried that I wanted the ordeal to be over now. I was so very tired. I just wanted it all to end. Why couldn't she wave some sort of wand and make it all go away, the pain, the humiliation and terrible shame, the nights of terror and the debilitating panic attacks? After all, that was the reason I came to this therapist in the first place. Now she was telling me that I would have to wait until my mind and my heart and the little girl inside me were ready to be joined. Not before would I get what I so desperately wanted. In that instant, I can honestly say I hated her. I thought that she was being horribly cruel, and I wanted to hurt her back. I discovered, however, that the choice was mine and the timing was mine. The more I tried to hurry, the slower the whole process became.

I found some degree of peace in going to yoga classes, and from having a reiki massage regularly. I began to realise that getting in touch with the divine energy within me through reiki and meditation were wonderful adjuncts to my healing. The power I found within myself stunned me. I began to realise that I was more powerful than the horrible memories and my stepfather, who is now old and weak. I think of it as the power of God. To me, it seems

as though that same power is the power Jesus used to heal people—
and it's in *me*. It was in the Little One all along. It's how she
managed to stay alive and not allow the monsters to kill her.

I still struggle with the shame, and the tendency to silence is
great. After all, the Little One lived with the threat of death for a
long time:

> I'm making my way to the top of the hole.
> My fingertips are almost able to reach the top—
> but not quite.
>
> I can see light. Do I want to see the light? Do I want it to
> see me?
> It may hurt me, it may burn me.
> It may enable others to see me.
> If they see me, really see me . . .
>
> I know this hateful hole, I've been in it for so long.
> I'm familiar with the rough and painful surface of its sides.
> I have begun to know where to find the jagged,
> bloodthirsty rocks,
> I can almost avoid them without looking.
>
> Am I succeeding?
> Is this progress?
> Is this the way out
>   or
> Just a fool's folly?
>
> Perhaps my fingertips are not as close to the top as I
> imagined.

I know that the Little One has survived; I have survived. Slowly,
I'm learning how to look after us and get out of that hole. After

all, what a terrible pity to have survived all that the Little One went through only to expire from neglect at my own hands. I remind myself every day that I am not bad, I'm good, and I'm a very special and talented woman. I eat small amounts now, I go to the gym, I take vitamins. I rest when I'm tired, I pray and I laugh, I cry, and I remind myself to really take in my beautiful family around me and enjoy every second of the time I have with them.

Sometimes I still mess up, but I can forgive myself those transgressions. The Little One is worth all the forgiveness and love in the world. She is precious. So are you all, God bless you.

Rowena Robinson

◆

Child abuse is a degrading, painful and humiliating experience. It takes hard, dedicated work and every atom of guts and willpower to achieve recovery, but there is life after abuse. You can make it to the top of the mountain, and when you do the view is breathtakingly lovely. I have never in my whole existence felt so empowered, so free. It's as if I could soar like an eagle among the peaks on every side.

Margaret Wood

HEALING THE SPIRIT

Most of us have found that there can be no ultimate healing without faith. We consider this element of our healing so important that we have made it a separate part of this healing chapter. For some, the church and organised religion have been connected with the abuse and it is difficult, but imperative for true healing, to separate the church and church dogma from true religion and our own faith—our belief in a higher power, the sense that we are all part of something greater than ourselves, and greater than the human species. Many of us call ourselves Christian, others Muslim or Hindu; others find it in nature or in a more general spiritual awareness affecting their lives. We believe that although people use different terms, and may have different affiliations and different interpretations, we are all, ultimately, talking about the same thing, and that it adds an extra—profound and vitally important—dimension to our healing. Those of us who are still here, fighting to heal, have not been destroyed by the evil which was imposed upon us because that inner light, our soul, has remained intact, pure and ready to guide us towards total healing.

One day when I was so sad and could contain it no longer I had a profound spiritual experience and I became aware that underneath all the pain and hurt there lay a deep love. I felt this love, which is within everyone—even our abusers, only in them it has been deeply buried.

Linda Honey

◆

Whenever I am centred I feel with God; whenever I dissociate, I am no longer with God and feel alone. God helps me to heal.

Lisa Patterson

◆

When I was most alone and facing up to what I knew would be my hardest memory to date, I prayed to God to be with me, to hold my hand and help me remember. He was, and so I had the strength to remember being raped. Afterwards I was filled, not with the normal exhausting remnants of emotions from my childhood, but with the most incredible sense of love. I knew then that God does care for us, and he is there in our hour of real need, if we just ask him for his help.

Liz Mullinar

◆

Spirituality is very much a personal thing. Many survivors feel an understandable mistrust of God, whatever they conceive him/her/

it to be. I was no exception. When I was 17 I joined the Pentecostal movement. Somehow, though, I never felt the cleansing or blessing of God. When I was 20 I developed the idea that he was going to give me cancer because I was so bad. Having no insight into the way my past had distorted my view of myself, this fear tormented me for two years, and only began to alleviate after some therapy, when that view began to be questioned.

For a long time I blamed God for my abuse. I felt he'd turned his back on me. I was angry. Healing for me has involved understanding that God cannot interfere with free will, even when it involves abuse of one of his precious children. But I believe he did do what he could. He gave me the spirit and strength to heal. He led me to people who assisted me.

For me spiritual healing also involved wiping the slate clean of some of the platitudes and concepts the church gave me, and asking God to reveal himself to me his way. His love is so beautiful. Some churches try to force the idea that you have to forgive and that your anger is a sin.

God does not force himself. I have an image of a God who was enraged by my abuse, and supports me as I move through my own anger. I hang on to the words of Jesus in St Mark's gospel: 'But whosoever causes one of these my little ones to stumble, it would be better for him if a millstone were hung around his neck and he were thrown into the sea.' Look out, my abusers!

As a feminist I was scared; I thought that God would want me to surrender my power to him, and become submissive, fearful and grovelling. The reality is, though, that he *added* to my sense of power. I feel so strong now, a feeling that wasn't there before I reached out to God. But he was only there when I was ready. God is not a spiritual rapist; he forces nothing, but guides my intuition. How I love him.

Louise Plummer

◆

Instead of externalising the inner struggle into blame and criticism of those around me, I am starting to take responsibility for my past and my responses. In knowing the unconditional love of an all-loving God I am able to love and forgive both myself and others. I am also coming to forgive those who hurt me—who, like me, are imperfect human beings. That is not to condone their actions but to realise that but for the grace of God, there go I. So while my life was once a daily struggle just to stay alive, now it is the quality of life I am concerned with. I move onwards hoping that one day, maybe, instead of hiding myself I will give of myself fully and unreservedly to the blessing and appreciation of others.

Joseph Elias

◆

My inner child is spiritually scarred as well as having been abused in other ways.

When a child goes to school it is given religious instruction. 'God is love,' Jesus said. 'Suffer the little children to come unto me.' But that child knows that at home God is not love, and Jesus has slammed the door in the child's face. So what is the child to believe?

In spite of the fact that I grew up in a religious household and school (we were dragged off to church every Sunday, and twice a day at school), the older I got the more disillusioned with the church I became. Finally I stopped believing altogether.

So it was with a sense of dawning wonder and joy that I was led back to spiritual beliefs: my discovery of a deeply Indian spiritual background, God, Jesus, higher power and my inner children.

Simon Williams

◆

Faith in God has been part of my life for 23 years now, ever since I was 13. When my husband died from cancer in August 1993 I knew he was with God and out of pain. Nature's numbness over the next few weeks kept me going. Then I started to feel pain beyond belief as I struggled to cope with my grief and with three girls all under the age of five.

My grief broke through the layers of protection I had built around myself, and I began another journey—to heal from multiple sexual abuse from family members. At a time when I desperately needed family support I was—and still am—very much alone. This shook my faith to the core. There have been so many questions about where I stand with God. Why did God, who is able to do anything, not stop my abuse or my husband's death? How could I reconcile my feelings of rejection and abandonment with a God who is supposed to be with me always? Is God's love trustworthy? Will God let me down?

My anger towards God has been intense, but as I gradually learn to put the blame where it really belongs, I am allowing his love to touch me bit by bit. I react strongly against the superficial answers that some churn out to people in crisis, but I can't deny God because I know in the depths of me that I am still here because of him. Most days all I can pray is that I will cope until the next.

My desire is that through this pain I will know the person of God, not just the traditions and expectations of believers around me. I believe there is an eternity for us all after this life. I take comfort in the fact that while I will be with God forever, my abusers will face a God of justice. This helps me to 'hang in there' with God. I am learning that God is different from those who hurt me so badly, and most of all that even within my current pain, the gospel of Jesus' death and resurrection out of love for us all, is true.

Anne Belling

✦

It must be my belief in something more powerful than myself. A sense that in time, if I continue to work hard, God will heal my brokenness. I do not believe that we are supposed to remain trapped within the pain of a damaged childhood. If possible we must seek to walk a personal path to the healing waters of life, a place where the sun shines on the inside of the soul, enabling the light of life to shine through the cracks of brokenness.

Jacinta McMurray

❖

Forgiveness came very late in the process of therapy (as it usually does). My mother had colluded with my father all through my years of childhood abuse (as well as abusing me herself for several years). I thought there was no way I could ever forgive her. Some years ago I had read a poem from Cathy Ann Matthews' book *Breaking Through*, which encouraged me to ask God to remove the blockages within me so that his forgiveness could flow through me to her. As I did that, amazing developments occurred. I had chosen not to speak of any memories with my mother (it was obvious she had buried them), so I verbalised my forgiveness towards her silently within myself.

Later I sent a beautiful brooch for Mother's Day as my token of forgiveness towards her. She rang to thank me warmly for the brooch. (I have always dutifully observed Mother's Day, but in a passive-aggressive fashion, i.e. I've usually chosen something fragile and sent it through the post hoping it would arrive broken!)

Our relationship has changed immeasurably. Mum cannot do enough for me, and I enjoy seeing her and seek opportunities to visit her. It is nothing short of a miracle. I am just so grateful to God for healing me and restoring my relationships in such an amazing and beautiful way.

June Harcourt

❖

Some days I want to shout for joy and run around stopping people to tell them: 'My trauma is over, it hardly seems possible, but it's true!' I'm so excited, so relieved, so grateful to my supporters and especially to God (who has heard and answered so many prayers), because I never thought I'd be able to say with such conviction that I am no longer dominated by the life-altering abuse I endured as a child. Now my days, my nights, my life are not controlled by the horrific memories or the on-going effects of the deep hurt and self-hatred that abusers impose, leaving their victims with habitually confusing, debilitating ways of thinking, acting and reacting.

Those pain-filled days, which had shackled my existence, have lost their power over my life. This hope for recovery I know is there for others who were abused, too. Don't misunderstand me. I'm not saying I have no problems; I'm not saying perhaps my abuse didn't happen. It happened, and its effects tormented my life for 50 years before I consciously remembered what my parents had done to me. When the memories returned I was racked by intense sorrow, pain, betrayed trust and hopelessness.

Inviting God to enter the depths of my violated spirit was difficult. I was so confused, had so many questions. Why didn't God help me? Where was God in all my suffering? I've often struggled to believe and pray. Now I had to find a way to trust him with these awful dilemmas and believe he could alleviate my suffering and lead me to spiritual recovery.

But how? Some might say I badgered God into helping me. (I guess I did, though now I know he intended me to.) I'd never have had the courage if my need hadn't been so intense. I knew that for me it had to be God that helped me or I'd never cope, never make it through. As I struggled to come to grips with the dichotomy between the horrors of my childhood and my belief that God loved me and cared about me, I finally admitted that behind my belief in God there was a great fear of him.

How does one approach a God one fears? As I queried this with God a verse leaped out at me from the Bible. Isaiah 43:26 says: 'Review the past for me . . . let us argue the matter together'.

What an offer! I reviewed, I argued—and I still do. I began to tell God as honestly as I could what I thought and felt about him, and this became the first of the steps to recovery. Surprisingly, pouring out this fear, blurting out my anger to God somehow gave me courage to move on and trust him more. It opened my eyes to the fact that I had equated God with my own unloving parents. But God and my parents are not the same.

Experiencing God's love gave me the courage to interact with him more fully. I could then tell him how badly I hurt, that I hated myself and thought I was worthless. This became my second step, the unburdening of my broken spirit to God. Working with God on steps three and four, asking him to amplify any results from my childhood that were hurting me or others now, opened my damaged spirit to his care and let me see each problem more clearly so I could ask God to manage me or overrule my reaction in whatever way he chose.

This step of overruling is a tricky one (and mighty unpopular) because it presupposes a trust in God that I do not always feel. Often I do not want him to take control of my life. But knowing that I cannot see every facet of my existence, and believing that God can, encourages me to ask him to overrule all my wants and desires. This can be pretty scary stuff, because I'm apprehensive that if he does overrule me I'll turn into a total doormat, a puppet person. Yet to my surprise the very opposite is taking place. God is constantly in the process of releasing and renewing the real me, rearranging my problems and bringing about my recovery. I cannot explain the process, I just know it is happening. God's spiritual solutions are enhancing my whole life.

I'm no longer the person I used to be. I've come a long way, acquired experience, learned many lessons, but not the ones to earn an academic degree. So I've awarded myself a degree: a BA for working and moving—Beyond Abuse.

One of the most confusing yet delightful steps I take is to acknowledge the presence of my inner child, who was me and still is me. She was the one who suffered so terribly, she is the one who needs recognition and comfort from both God and me. When

I was molested my reactions were huge and life-changing. I was sure that there was something very very wrong with me when someone could choose to hurt me and no one else even seemed to care. This was a totally wrong assumption; the fault for my abuse was not and is not mine. Over the years I've learnt to love my inner child Cathy (little me). I've come to see how beautiful she is, how amazingly brave she has been, and that God loves her and me very dearly. I've chosen to stop hating her and treating her badly as others did.

We can choose to let God work or we can pull back, still afraid, still torn by our own internal opposition to him, which can keep us in a state of confusion and resistance. We can begin to see that as much as we long to be in control of our own lives, we cannot be. This is a human desire that it's impossible to fulfil. So we can take our courage in both hands and ask God to be the one who controls our lives.

Gradually this can lead us into my final step: I choose to forgive. It's my last step, because so much needs to be worked through before we can even begin to think about forgiving our abusers and ourselves. So much growing and changing before we even want to forgive. Perhaps we will not want to forgive, but we do have the option to choose to be willing to forgive. This then sets into action a dynamic I do not even begin to understand. But I know the reality of it. I know, without a doubt, that God works in a special way if I am willing to choose to forgive. It enables God's love and all the benefits of giving and accepting forgiveness to flow freely out through each of our relationships in an ever-widening circle.

We who have suffered the damaging effects of abuse all need God. And he, I believe, longs to help us, especially in our deep spiritual suffering—if we will let him.

Cathy Ann Mathews

◆

There is something there, some spirit (not necessarily a spirit), something within life, an inner dynamic, vitality. I have this 'faith', feel this something striving, searching, from beyond the dark abyss I was plunged into.

This darkness is not my life. I try to find this 'realness', this 'something'. I cannot find it in their eyes in school, in church, in university, in the work places, at parties, even at the quiet talking moments—it is so often not there, or only glimpsed for a fleeting moment.

It is there in the trees, the sunrise and the sunset, the moon, the stars, the river, the animals, insects, fungi, the genuine ... everything. Pushed to the very edge of nothingness, I refuse to give in, to my last breath I know there is something.

Struggling in the pit, on the edge of death—so many times—I am finding the way. Finding this something. Finding the genuine heart in relationship, taking a new look at the new, awe-inspiring beauty of nature and also my own part within this nature, within Life.

John Tardy

✦

I had worked as a Christian nurse overseas for some years before beginning therapy. Throughout the years of therapy my relationship with God was a very unpredictable one. As therapy began I felt utterly cut off from everyone, including God. My whole world was turned upside down. I felt I was adrift with no moorings. For some years I even doubted that God could exist, yet inwardly I longed for his love and comfort to be a reality. As I progressed through very difficult episodes in therapy, I began to meet regularly with my church minister, who prayed for my healing. He accepted me wherever I was at in my relationship with God. Loving friends also supported and enabled me to experience God's love and care. Gradually, healing came. Now the struggle is over, and I have a different—warm and loving—relationship with God. I can be

open and honest with him in a way that before therapy was foreign
to me.

June Harcourt

◆

PLEASE GOD

The drive in the car makes me feel all this pain.
Is it just 'cause I'm older he chooses my body?
Please God, don't let it happen again.

We've arrived. I tremble. We greet 'him' again.
His movements remind me of each previous crime.
So deep in my heart I am sure it's my fault.
Please God, don't let it happen this time.

My mummy, my daddy, I love them so much,
But I can't let them know that there's something amiss.
I can't be that honest; they'll no longer love me.
Please God, don't let it happen like this.

He's there. I'm afraid. How I hate this moment.
He gets me alone. I just feel I could die.
I'm a bad boy. I must be, for him to do it.
Please, God, why is it me, oh why?

I feel so dirty; the guilt and the shame.
It's an endless fall down a bottomless pit.
I can't help that I'm young. What can I do?
God, I'm so angry! Just make him quit.

I can't tell Mummy, I can't tell Daddy.
I can't tell anyone, can't tell at all.
I just can't trust them to know my secret.

Please God, help me to block my recall.

It makes me feel that I'm such a bad person.
Whenever we visit, it's just like before.
How in the world can a little boy cope?
Please God, help me to feel good once more.

After so many years trying not to feel it,
I see him as desperate, see pain in his past.
Let my heart feel the strength of sincere forgiveness;
Find the love I can feel for myself, at last.

Brian Bell

◆

One morning I went to a park, and finding it hard to clear my mind to pray, decided to write my prayer. One question I asked with great intensity was, 'God, where were you when I was being abused?'

In just a few moments I found myself writing down the answer: 'I was there with you feeling your pain'. This touched me so deeply I wept tears of relief—God did love me, he hadn't abandoned me!

I've held on to that comfort, but have continued to have fights with God. During times of intense pain I have asked, 'Where is God in all this?'

The times I've felt most cared for and closest to God have been when I've been prayed for by my therapist or a trusted friend. As I continue to deal with the effects on my life of the sexual abuse I suffered, my relationship with God is being tested every inch of the way. I feel I want to hold at a distance this God who I've known for most of my life. He is my father who loves, who is sovereign, yet he judges, he allows suffering. My father also loved me, he had control over me. I suffered, I was at his mercy. At one point I wanted nothing to do with this remote-seeming God—then I remembered Jesus. I love the Jesus of the gospels—compassionate, a healer, he was concerned for the outcasts of society, he touched the leper, spent time caring for and talking with women; yet, being human, he felt tired, stressed, lonely and rejected.

From time to time during therapy I've had the image of myself as a child, firmly held in Jesus's arms. He loved children. He understands. He was human—he was abused, betrayed, stripped, beaten, exposed, nailed, hung to die, abandoned by God and by his friends.

He understands.

I go to church every Sunday; my little church is an extension of my family. I have shared my story only with a few. More Sundays than not in that first year I sat with tears pouring down my cheeks. No one noticed or, if they did, they chose not to mention it to me. Mostly the service wasn't helpful, but at times I would be touched by the words and music of a song.

My therapist shared with me an idea she had had for some time—a worship service planned for survivors. She also suggested the names of a few women who would also be interested and, after much initial indecision on on my part, I took the initiative and contacted these women and we organised a task force to plan the service. At last (seven months later!) the service was held. It was a truly special event. It was attended by over 200 people and we had a great deal of positive feedback—survivors did not feel so alone; we had a sense that the church *did* care. It was okay to express our feelings in a worship context. It's okay to argue with God. There is hope—we can experience healing and we can minister to each other.

My spiritual struggles still continue. I often wish God were more tangible, real. I want to experience the feeling of being in Jesus's arms—not just to imagine it. God and I are still friends. I know it's okay with him for me to be wherever I'm at. I continue to worship and serve him and learn more about him, and I'm even open to desiring a closer relationship with him. Ultimately, I am his.

Joy P. Gordon

✦

I've prayed for years that God would do a miraculous healing in my life. The closest thing to this happened recently. Suddenly— and I mean suddenly—as I was driving my car home from having coffee with a friend, it hit me: it doesn't matter what I was like as a child, even if I was strong-willed, naughty, grumpy—whatever, I didn't deserve what happened to me. I know this knowledge was from God. Only a week earlier I had cancelled my appointments with my counsellor. I just kept hitting brick walls. I couldn't get past blaming myself—if only I hadn't been naughty, or bad, or impatient.

Whatever I was as a child, it was because of my surroundings. This miracle has given me the courage to face issues I couldn't even acknowledge before. Just knowing God is there, even though I still question his abandoning me as a child, has helped me to believe there is hope. I don't have to be a victim. I don't have to be who they (my family) made me—God can make me new.

Juley Taben

✦

I have an inkling that God is deeper than my pain, my horror, my fear.

Anne Belling

✦

Knowing in your heart and soul that you are special—unique— can be a long time coming for a person who has lived through the trauma of abuse. Accepting it can take even longer. However, I believe we are called by God (who loves us unconditionally) to claim, name and live in our specialness, our uniqueness, as a part of the creation in which we are everyday participants. Our uniqueness is what makes us special, because there is no other person exactly like us on this planet. Who we are, our life experiences (both good and bad) are what makes us the original, distinctive, unique person that each of us is, both in the eyes of the world and in the eyes of God.

Stephanie Casey

✦

I used to feel so dreadfully cut off from God. And when I prayed, I felt I hardly ought to, because I was such a fraud. I didn't deserve contact with God. I couldn't pray right—I just didn't qualify for inclusion. But with the hell of drinking again staring me in the face, I prayed anyway.

My counsellor, Bill, put to me that God is to do with 'infinite acceptance'. Of course I wanted this to be true, but it so went against what was inside me—the enormous inability to accept myself or conceive that anyone else would.

Over the years, a deeply negative image of God has remained, and great reluctance to put myself in his care. My sense of it, strongly, is of being grovelly, submissive to some unloving, domineering and controlling male being, one who is considered ever so separate and superior. Despite what I've heard over the years, or even what I think, this has remained my feeling sense of God. To avoid this, I don't think of God as a being at all.

It doesn't take much to figure out what I'd like God to be—loving, accepting and interested. I have trouble thinking in terms of 'me and God' at all. It only heightens the keen sense of separation that I have. It's helped me to talk with a friend who also has difficulty with God. I can look at her and see how hard she tries. Sharing with her has helped me feel less bad.

I've felt a lot of anger towards God over the years. I'm not even sure why. Maybe I feel abandoned, and resent the superior 'I'm never wrong' position that always leaves me taking the blame for things. I've imagined God standing smugly to one side while I take the rap. Gee, I resent that—God made me!

Something I've come to realise for myself is that what really counts is to be kind to others—a major lifetime's undertaking. There's lots of learning in it. Other people's caring and kindness and time is what has got me through my most difficult moments— the many times I've felt suicidal, or felt like drinking, or just got so keenly distressed by my feelings. I've wandered around the psychiatric hospital, marvelling that these people think I'm worth saving.

Once, a nurse was saying how strong she thought my spirit was. I cursed my strong spirit, and promptly burst into tears. Who wanted to stay alive to go through *this*? I could imagine God understanding and laughing gently.

These days I'm doing pretty well, and can feel my heart opening up. This is very exciting—the main event—and it makes me feel whole. Who cares if I'm a bit crazy? I think I've come a long way. I no longer live in torment, I can relate to others quite well, and I'm happy to be alive. I no longer feel like drinking—a major miracle. I feel like kissing the ground and saying, 'Thank you, God'.

Maybe I'm not doing so bad on the God front after all. I have a lot more self-acceptance, which is like heaven on earth. And that extreme sense of self-blame and criticism—where has it gone? Another miracle.

Music has been a great way for me to get a sense of God. Sometimes it has been the only way. One time in hospital, I was in acute anxiety with my first realisations of severe abuse. I played some Chopin on my Walkman, desperate for anything to calm me down. It was beautiful music, and in the middle of it I got a sense of God. This sense was of God as totally unassuming and innocent, gentle, playful, passionate, and very much interested in me.

This really took me by surprise. It's good to remember this

image now. I also have a vague idea that what's deepest in me, in my own nature, is of God, that there's no separation at all.

My mind feels very alive, and that's not of my own making. Even the efforts I make are not really 'mine'. There's just some kind of inner flow—I was born, not self-made.

There have been quite a few miracles in my life—and probably some I don't recognise. I think lots has happened without my being aware of it. If there was a reason I wanted to live, it was for the chance to express some loving. At this point in time I feel whole and rich—I just want to share it! I still need people, and caring is a need for others too.

Wendy Nelson

◆

I stood waiting to be served communion as the flashback hit.

My first communion day. It was so special: I was seven years old and dressed all in white. As I approached the altar I was engulfed in shame, but I could not turn back so I took the communion.

I returned to my seat. 'So dirty, so dirty. God does not want dirty people here. Dirty people do not take Holy Communion. What will God do to me? He will punish me for this.' Terrible fear was added to my shame.

The flashback was awful. I stood there shaking. Silent tears dripped off my chin onto my silk shirt. Then something happened. In my mind I saw Jesus crucified: not as religious art, because that always showed him wearing a loincloth. He was on the cross naked, as he had been crucified.

In my mind I could hear the soldiers mocking his genitals. Then with great clarity, I recalled that during times of intense fear and pain, the sphincter lets go. Somehow I saw the immense shame and degradation that Jesus felt, and I realised how much greater his shame was than the shame I had experienced in the flashback.

I was served the communion emblems: the remembrance of the death of Jesus Christ. As I took the bread and wine, somehow, in a way that's difficult to explain, I gave my shame in exchange for them. It was unforgettable: the shame was gone.

As I continue to work through my recovery, at times I experience intense emotional pain. I still ask the same question: how could any human being subject another human to such sadistic degradation? Its depths seem limitless. It is often difficult to face another day; the question is always in my mind: what horrors will today bring? However, whatever arises, I am now able to face it without the added weight of the shame. It has not been repressed; it no longer lives. My shame has gone, and I *know* it.

Mary S.

◆

It's hard to describe the inner world that I found while I was healing. I'd long had an image of a dark room at the bottom of a winding staircase. At the far side there was a door, slightly open. There was light the other side of the door, and I wanted to go through it, or at least to open the door wider to let in more light. When I first tried to meditate I would find myself in this room. It seemed that whatever lay on the other side of the door was important, but despite my feeling of longing, I could not 'go' there.

Since I've rescued my little child, and she has integrated with my spirit self, my innate wisdom, I've been able to move through the (now wide open) doorway. It leads to another world, a world without end, in which all is light and love. It is so light there are no shadows, for the light is all around. Whenever I focus on healing, I go through the door. I am aware of a presence that is everywhere, is all-encompassing, unknowable, infinite and eternal. If I wait, and especially if I think of awe and gladness, if I 'lift up my heart', I become filled with the warmth of the light and the love; it is like being bathed in inner sunlight. There's also a sense of welcome and delight, and my awe contains no fear and much joy. It is a place of peace and rest and refreshment.

Sometimes I'm aware of a great reluctance to return to 'this world' from the place of light, which feels like home. Then I am gently nudged, and reminded that I belong in this world too, for now. It's impossible to describe what being on 'the other side' is like, except in clichés: it's a place of perfect peace, where I am fully known, where there is no struggle or pain because Love is all. I don't understand it (though it understands me!), and that doesn't matter. I know it is to do with grace, and belief, and with being a part of a spiritual universe, and that to have been shown it is a profoundly important gift. More than anything else, I know that this is where my healing lies.

Candida Hunt

◆

COME AND SKIP
His back was firm and wide
and as he turned towards her,
she thought she sensed deep love, acceptance
and compassion in the depths of his eyes.
He laughed and simply said
'Come and skip with me'.
The child within flew like an arrow true into his arms,
and as they embraced their eyes met
and they laughed together.
They turned and looked towards this woman,
and both said, 'Come and skip'.

She remembered other enticing invitations
that ended in humiliation,
pain and rape—the betrayal of a father, brother, mother.

The pain was raw, having taught her not to trust,
not to accept enticing invitations,

but as she looked deep within her,
something deeper stirred.
It bubbled and convulsed
through layers of pain, betrayal, lust and hate,
until she held it gently in her hand.
She had found a seed of love, hope and trust.

She looked towards the man and child,
and keeping her eyes fixed on him,
She began to deliberately place one foot in front of the
    other,
as she walked towards them.

Sometimes the seed within her grew,
at other times it seemed to disappear altogether.
The journey was fearsome, racked with pain.
Sometimes filled with anger and rage
She raged, screamed and cried,
other times so despondent she curled in a ball wanting to
    die.

Still, eyes on him, she walked,
she begged for an acceptable disease to take her out,
so the family would not have to bear the label suicide.

In his church she could count those who accepted her
on the fingers of one hand.
The more she looked the more it seemed
the church was on the side of injustice.
It was immersed in platitudes,
it lived the 'victorious life' and had no time for struggle
    and pain.
Cynicism was born, as she saw his compassion
and the church's inability to move in integrity

to the side of the oppressed and hurt
it covered over the sins of abuse within its walls.

Still she walked, her eyes on him,
and all the while racing around the perimeter of her mind
was the word 'crazy, crazy, crazy',
don't believe this, it can't be true.

Yet deep inside, the child looked with large and pain-filled
    eyes:
'Believe it happened, it is the truth within you,
but needs to come into the light',
and on she walked, her eyes on him.

She met them, the child and the Son of God,
and placed her hands in theirs.
They turned and walked into the cloud that was their
    future,
and held gently within the embrace of the three
was the woman's deep longing to skip,
and deep within herself she knew she would
and on she walked, her eyes on him.

Cherry Bavinton

✦

I am a spiritual being. I identify with spirit. I have experienced such awe, joy and love on this level, and I have experienced such pain and despair on the human level.

My abuse began when I was only three months old. It was dreadful, but there were gifts in the experiences I had. Because I was so young when the abuse began, I never became fully grounded in my physical body; my being was able to remain identified with the spiritual part of myself. Some would call this dissociation, but for me the two states are different. The way I am on a spiritual level feels very different from what happens when I am dissociating.

All through my childhood I identified with nature, and when I attended church services—and particularly around Christmas and Easter—the tears would stream down my face and I would feel awe and grief. I do not identify with being a Christian or a member of any other religion; I identify with the state of grace sometimes called universal love or love energy. Experiencing this state of grace seems to depend on me: when I am quiet, and not using busyness or addictive substances I am able to be aligned with the spiritual part of myself. At other times it can be very difficult to have the contact.

The gifts of spirit, love and forgiveness are a direct result of the abuse from my father. There were times when my memories were coming back that I was suicidal, and didn't want to believe the pain in me. But because of this spiritual awareness, I was able to sink fully into the pain and come out the other side with courage, strength and peace. It gave me the ability to detach and trust my healing process, and to see and know that all things, even the pain, are ultimately for my highest good and greatest joy. Out of what most people would say were impossible issues to heal from have come my greatest learning and greatest letting go, the importance of focusing on my truth, and lastly that my father was my greatest enemy and at the same time my greatest gift, because he gave me the awareness of things beyond the reality that we normally see.

Through these experiences I know my truth and the reality of who I really am: a spiritual being who is a survivor of childhood physical and sexual abuse.

Deane Griffin

◆

Four years ago last September
I started out on a journey.

I didn't want anyone to see me.
I didn't like being noticed,
I felt everyone would see how bad I was.
But over the years,
As I began unpacking the truth of my childhood
And finding the horror, pain, shame, guilt and fear
That I carried,
Ever so slowly my awareness began to grow,
And there came faith and understanding
That the things I had unpacked
Belonged to those who had caused them
In the child me.
I look at myself with different eyes now,
Still striving to grow and heal
And to be a part of the here and now.
And now it doesn't really matter
Whether others notice me or not.
There is a sense of well-being inside me,
A connectedness to this world and beyond.

Sally Bateman

◆

When I was ten years old my mother failed to protect me from abuse by a family friend. I came to feel very guilty about the feelings of hate I had towards her, because I knew God wouldn't want me to feel like this.

When I was 45 I went on a course where I spent half the time in lectures and the other half learning how to put Christian counselling into practice. Part of the experience was to be counselled myself so that I wouldn't bring my own baggage into a counselling session. Trainees are expected to deal with any problems in their primary care relationships, with partners or with their children.

By the time my sessions were over, I felt like a new person. It was nothing short of a miracle. All my feelings of hurt, anger, shame, guilt and rejection were healed, for God had taken all these burdens from me as he promises to do. On the way home, I felt the spirit of God telling me to forgive my mother and say sorry for my part in our bad relationship. I did, explaining to her how I felt that God had healed me, and asking her to forgive me as I had forgiven her. I reached out to hug her, but she remained frozen. Over the next few weeks I tried to reach her in love, but she was always negative. I used to feel angry about this, but I think she had to learn to trust me again. I noticed a softening in her attitude after about six months, and we began to be a little more open with each other. We are closer now, and I have grown to love her. I believe God changed my heart, and that made the difference.

I want to encourage everyone not to give up. God can help you to restore broken relationships. It takes time. It takes effort. It takes commitment. But it's worth it.

Margaret Eyre

◆

I always knew the storm would pass. I didn't know how long it would last or how fierce it might blow, but as I sit here now and reflect, I realise I just knew, intuitively, that maybe if I didn't panic, didn't feel the pain, didn't run, it would pass.

I just accepted that on 'those' occasions when the monster entered our house, I could always tell by the manner in which the door was opened, the heaviness of the footstep, the immediate tightening of my spirit, what lay ahead. No, that's wrong. I (we) never knew what lay ahead, and I suppose that was the fear. I have since discovered, with guidance from those who have gained knowledge and awareness, that 'the fear within us is far greater than any fear before us'. Knowing this is the foundation of my recovery, my ability to conquer my fears.

I loved my father then, as I love him now. As a child I could not understand what made him lash out at the very ones who loved him, and who I knew he also loved. I am my father's son. I carried the same fears as him, the dysfunctional feelings. I had no other role model, so the cycle continued for another 30 years. I then found my answer: I had to let go. I had to truly accept a higher power. I had to find faith—faith in who I am, not the fears of lost spirit but the true acceptance of living in the now, a day at a time. Having the absolute belief that nothing happens by chance, that the journey and how we conduct ourselves, our motives, our principles, are what it is about. Not to blame others, but to accept, to understand that we humans are multi-layered, extraordinary creatures, and that the only person we exercise any control over is ourself.

Tony Bonner

◆

It seems that often the deeper the pain and trauma, the greater the spirituality. For some survivors, the connection with the light, or with angelic beings, or with a divine energy, was the only joy or support that was felt throughout the abuse: for some it was what helped them to survive, was the only source of help or sense of love in a dark and painful world.

In therapy it seems that the survivors who discover a strong sense of spirituality are the ones for whom the healing process is a journey, the ones who have a strong incentive to keep going even when all the odds seem to be against them. For some, only healing of a spiritual nature is able to touch the core of their shattered soul, and to facilitate their progress through the emotional and physical pain.

I wonder if it is possible to find our spiritual self without going on a journey of pain and suffering? I believe that spirituality and wounding are in a dance together: that each is energetically bound to the other, and that without the experience of the wounding, the soul would lack the impetus to search for the truth. And without this search, would we ever come to our spiritual self?

For the therapist working with survivors of childhood abuse, spirituality has a dual function. The first is as a guiding force in the healing process itself, which may link in with the survivor's awareness, and the second is for the therapist—to help cope with the horror and pain of clients' traumas, as well as acting as a preventive measure against the effects of burnout and vicarious traumatisation.

So we have a therapeutic relationship, which is enhanced by each person's spirituality—regardless of its nature—and the therapeutic process, which is enhanced by an added dimension and awareness. Little or much may be spoken on the subject, yet the effects are all-encompassing and are a positive force for healing. And isn't healing the whole person what therapy is ultimately about? Bringing the body, the mind, the emotions and the spirit into harmony?

Zoe Hagon

♦

Through the sobs forcing their way up through the pain-filled layers of fear and self-hate came the words, 'My father stole all that was me'.

During the long and difficult counselling process, I slowly began to realise that in fact my father had not stolen 'all that was me'. I had instead needed to hide it deep within me, away from my father and even from myself. I also began to see that if this were so, then I could be in control of reclaiming myself. This is how the healing process began.

I gradually became aware that I was not alone. There was someone else with me, willing me into the reclamation of my wholeness. This someone I chose to name God. My God, who I realised was already within me, who had always been there with me, in my pain, terror and confusion. This God had grieved with me, raged with me, cried with me and experienced the same powerlessness with me, and always, always valued and loved me.

I began to understand that God was loving me into my on-going healing. I discovered, through questioning and challenging, that God could be trusted never to be invasive or intrusive, would always wait to be invited, never forced anything, was a God who was constant and patient, was waiting for me, calling to me, loving me.

I began to know that there was, deep within me, a core from which came the knowledge that I was okay, that what happened to me was real, that I was not to blame. The many tears of rage and pain I shed came from that core part, which knew and trusted my own reality, and knew the rightness of my memories and the wrongness of my father's deeds. I also came to know that at the deepest centre of my core was my God.

As I learned to trust God, I began to see that if God loved me so much—all of me, every little bit of me—then maybe, just maybe, I could let God teach me to love myself in the way that God does. I am in partnership with God in the process of reclaiming 'all that was me'. I can never be alone on my journey.

As told to Shona Margaret Chisholm

✦

'There is no difficulty that enough love will not conquer. There is no disease that enough love will not heal. No door that enough love will not open. No gulf that enough love will not bridge. No wall that enough love will not throw down. And no sin that enough love will not redeem. It makes no difference how deeply seated may be the trouble. How hopeless the outlook. How muddled the tangle. How great the mistake. A sufficient realisation of love will dissolve it all. And if you could love enough you would be the happiest and most powerful person in the world.'

Emmett Fox, quoted by Louise L. Hay in The Power is Within You

✦

APPENDIX 1

THE ASCA STORY

ASCA—Advocates for Survivors of Child Abuse—is a non-profit organisation dedicated to helping adult men and women come to terms with their childhood trauma. It was founded in 1995 by psychologist Dr Martha C. Dean, Pauline Groves, Liz Mullinar and Christopher Thomson to provide a voice for survivors.

ASCA focuses on healing, because without healing, life for survivors is a test of endurance without relief, without peace and without the possibility of true happiness.

ASCA is a national organisation with informal social groups operating in all states. We believe that contact with other survivors is a vital part of the healing process. We believe that survivors, better than anyone else, understand our own needs.

Being a member of ASCA helps dispel the feelings of being alone in the pain of an abusive past. Members benefit from the understanding of other members, by discovering that there is no need to bury shame and other difficult feelings deep inside, and that the road to healing begins by opening outwards. This book is, in itself, a part of the healing process of our members.

ASCA services include a monthly newsletter; a resource centre with books, tapes, videos etc; a national referral list of therapists who are experienced with adult survivors; and a 24-hour phone support line.

We warmly invite you to join us. Everyone knows the cold statistics of child abuse, but by translating mere numbers into real people with a powerful voice, we believe we can effect meaningful social change.

ASCA
PO Box 842
Darlinghurst NSW 2010
Tel: 02 9360 7281
Tel/fax: 02 9331 2487
FREECALL 1800 657 380

Donations to ASCA are tax-deductible.

APPENDIX 2

ORGANISATIONS FOR SURVIVORS

We have not listed any sexual assault services as most of them do not provide services for adult survivors of child sexual assault. Check with your local SAS to see if they can help you.

ASCA (Advocates for Survivors of Child Abuse)
PO Box 842
Darlinghurst NSW 2010
Tel: 02 9360 7281
Tel/fax: 02 9331 2487
FREECALL 1800 657 380

Australian Association of Trauma & Dissociation
PO Box 85
Brunswick VIC 3056
Tel: 03 9663 6225
Fax: 03 9639 4881

Beyond Survival
This is a bi-monthly magazine on ritual abuse, trauma and dissociation.
For information ring (02) 9566 2046 or write to
Beyond Survival
PO Box 85
Annandale NSW 2038

Broken Rites
for any male or female abused by the church (any denomination)
PO Box 163
Rosanna VIC 3084
Tel: 03 9457 4999 (Contact: Bernard)

Dissociative Identity Society of South Australia
PO Box 440
Parkholme SA 5043

Incest Survivors' Association Inc.
21 Lacey Street

East Perth WA 6004
Tel: 09 227 8745
Fax: 09 227 1510

Men Against Sexual Assault (MASA)
PO Box 1208
Darlinghurst NSW 2010
Tel: 02 9360 7613

Men Against Sexual Assault (MASA)
PO Box 26
ACT 2602
Tel: 06 247 9227

Merging All Parts (MAP) Inc.—Dissociative Identity Disorder Support
Group
PO Box 1163
Penrith NSW 2751
Tel: 047 31 3309
A self-help support group for people diagnosed as experiencing
dissociation and/or Dissociative Identity Disorder (DID) and their
supporters.

Rainbow Male Survivors Network
PO Box 2186
Richmond South VIC 3121
Tel: 03 9421 0446
Fax: 03 9510 5699
e-mail: rainbownet@yarranet.au
website: http://yarranet.net.au/rmsn/rainbownet.htm
A gay support group.

RASS (Ritual Abuse Survivors and Supporters)
Sydney: PO Box 63, Camperdown NSW 2050
Wollongong: PO Box 5379, Wollongong NSW 2500
Melbourne: PO Box 5, Dingley VIC 3172
Western Victoria: PO Box 485, Stawell VIC 3380
Tel: 053 581 343
Adelaide: c/- North Adelaide Women's Community Health Centre, 64
Pennington Terrace, North Adelaide SA 6005

Uniting Survivors and Supporters
c/- Friendship House
20 Balfour Street
New Farm QLD 4005
Tel: 07 3358 4988

VOICES
WA group for those abused by the Christian Brothers
Contact: Bruce Blythe
PO Box 81
Como WA 6152
Tel: 09 421 1034 (work) or 09 450 2513 (home)

Women Incest Survivors Network
PO Box 370
Leichhardt NSW 2040
Tel: 02 9560 6627
Membership of WISN is open to all female survivors of incest and
child sexual assault.

Other organisations
New South Wales
The Women's Centre
63 Tudor Street
Belmore NSW 2192
Tel: 02 9718 1955
Individual and group counselling for adult survivors.

Child Protection Enforcement Agency
02 9286 7276

Male Sexual Assault Services
Eastern and Central Sexual Assault Services
Level 5, Building 72
Royal Prince Alfred Hospital
Missenden Road, Camperdown NSW 2050
Tel: 02 9515 7566

Dympna House
Counselling and resource centre for CSA (women only and no ritual
abuse survivors)

PO Box 22 Haberfield NSW 2045
Tel: 02 9797 6733
Fax: 02 9799 6095

Sydney Rape Crisis Centre
02 9819 6565 or 9819 7842
1800 424 017 (within NSW, outside Sydney)
24 hour counselling line and information about other services for
survivors.

Rosie's Place
PO Box 40
Rooty Hill NSW 2766
PH: 02 9625 2599
Provides counselling for males/females up to 18 years old and groups
for mothers whose children have been abused.

Australian Capital Territory
Domestic Violence Crisis Service
PO Box 320
Civic Square ACT 2601
Tel: 06 248 7800

Canberra Rape Crisis Centre
PO Box 813
Dickson ACT 2602
Tel (administration): 06 247 8071
Fax: 06 247 2536
Crisis counselling line: 06 247 2525 (24 hrs)
06 247 1657 TTY (9-5; leave message)

Victoria
Domestic Violence and Incest Resource Centre (DVIRC)
DVIRC is a state-wide service in Victoria which offers counselling,
information and resources (videos, books, training) to victims of
domestic violence and incest. DVIRC is open from
9 to 5 Monday to Friday.
Public telephone line: 03 9387-9155
Administration line: 03 9380-4343
Fax: 03 9380-4373

WIRE (Women's Information & Referral Exchange)
Tel: 03 9654 6844

Australians Against Child Abuse (AACA)
PO Box 525
Ringwood VIC 3134
Tel: 03 9870 6261
Fax: 03 9879 6148
Counselling for children up to age 17.

CASA (Centre Against Sexual Assault)
270 Cardigan Street Carlton VIC 3053
Crisis line: 03 9344 2210
Administration line: 03 9347 3066
Fax: 03 9347 1505
Counselling lines: 03 9349 1766 or 1800 806 292 (if you live outside
metropolitan Melbourne)
Branches in Ballarat, Bendigo, East Bentleigh, East Ringwood,
Footscray, Geelong, Heidelberg, Horsham, Mildura, Morwell,
Parkville, Shepparton, Wangaratta, Warrnambool. 24-hour crisis care
services, counselling and group work.

Queensland
Rape and Incest Counselling—24 hour support line
Tel: 07 3844 4008
Provide face-to-face court support as well as counselling

Cairns Rape Crisis Centre (24 hrs)
Tel: 070 313 590
Telephone (men and women) and face-to-face (women) counselling for
adult survivors.

Sunshine Coast Crisis Centre
Tel: 074 434 334 or 1800 012 023 (Qld country) (9–5, weekdays
only)

Tablelands Women's Sexual Assault Service
Tel: 070 912 334 (24 hr)

Women's Info Link
Tel: 07 3229 1264

Women's Health Centre
Tel: 07 3839 4988

South Australia
Rape & Sexual Assault Services
Tel: 08 8226 8777 (9–5) or 1800 817 421 (SA only)
Have counselling for both male and female survivors.

Crisis Care Counselling (SA only)
131 611 (after 4pm)

Women's Statewide Health Services
08 8267 5366 (9–5, M–F)

Men's Contact and Resource Centre
PO Box 8036
Hindley Street
Adelaide SA 5000
Tel: 08 223 1110

Positive Action Centre for Survivors of Abuse (PACSA)
North Adelaide SA 5???
Tel: 08 8239 0177

Western Australia
Sexual Assault Referral Centre
PO Box 842
Subiaco WA 6008
Tel: 09 340 1828 (8.30–5 weekdays) or 09 964 1853 (crisis care 24hrs) or 1800 199 888 (WA country)

Port Hedland Sexual Referral Centre
PO Box 93
Port Hedland WA 6721
Tel: 091 73 3337 (24 hours)

Eastern Goldfield Sexual Assault Referral Centre
PO Box 1373
Kalgoorlie WA 6430
Tel: 090 91 1922 (24 hours)

Tasmania
Sexual Assault Support Service
PO Box 217
North Hobart TAS 7002
Tel: 002 31 1811 (24 hours)

Laurel House
PO Box 1062
Launceston TAS 7250
Tel: 003 34 2740 (9–5; after hours: 016 181450 paging service)

Northern Territory
Darwin Centre Against Rape
Ruby Gaea House
Tel: 08 8945 0155 (9–5, weekdays only)

Sexual Assault Referral Centre
Tel: 089 22 7156

APPENDIX 3

SETTING UP A SELF-HELP GROUP

Self-help groups can provide a welcome source of support for survivors. If you are thinking of setting one up, there are several things that will help to make the group helpful and successful.

Organising the group

Self-help groups do not have a professional leader and are not facilitated: the group members themselves shape the group to meet their needs. All members are equal, and any expertise within the group is there for everyone to share. One important message to get across is that each member will have input on the running of the group. This helps to ensure that everyone feels safe, and encourages members to realise their own strengths without any one member being chosen to act as a dominant focus.

Venue

You will need to find a safe, easily accessible and comfortable place to meet. It could be one group member's home, several members' homes in turn, or a room that can be loaned or rented. Community cottages, neighbourhood centres and other organisations may be able to offer you space for meetings.

The advantages of renting a meeting room are that it is neutral ground for everyone, and will always be available on the dates you arrange. The cost may prove a disadvantage.

The advantage of using a group member's home is that it will be free and won't feel institutional. The disadvantages might include the feeling that the host member is set apart—others may feel uncomfortable, and so may the host. If the same home is the venue, that member may feel burdened because they always have to be available (even if they are ill, etc.).

Costs and funding

Members will need to pay for rent (perhaps), and cover the cost of tea/coffee and other refreshments, any materials the group may wish to purchase or publish, postage, etc. You will need to decide what to charge for membership, bearing in mind that people's financial situation may not be easy. Keep your costs as low as possible.

Some local councils have small amounts of funding available to assist in setting up a group. Other local organisations may also be able to help. Don't be afraid to ask: the worst anyone can do is turn you down!

Who's in charge

One member will need to keep track of the group's finances, look after any property, and organise meeting dates, etc. This could be arranged in rotation so that each member can benefit from the responsibility, or the tasks could be shared out among members according to what contribution people feel able to make to the group as a whole.

The responsibility of being the group leader can be very challenging; members need to be aware of the struggles they may face.

Advertising and contacts

In order to attract new members to the group you will need to decide on how best to publicise the group's existence, and how potential members may contact the group. Advertising individual members' telephone numbers may not be a good idea: you could receive cranky or hostile calls, and also calls from men or women in crisis. As a self-help group you are not qualified to deal with these—though it is a good idea to have an extensive list of helpful phone contacts to pass on to a caller.

It may be preferable for the group to buy an answering machine and ensure that it is regularly checked, and to share the task of calling people back. It may also be possible for an organisation, neighbourhood centre, etc. to screen calls and pass on details of genuine enquiries to you.

Type of group

Different survivors have different needs. What kind of group will yours be: women only, men only or mixed; heterosexual only, gay/lesbian only; any age barriers (child, teenage and adults needs are very different)? These are just a few examples. It is important to think about these things to ensure that the group does not fragment because people do not have enough in common.

You will also need to decide whether the group will be a closed group or open to new members on a drop-in basis.

Group rules

This may seem a bit formal, but without a set of agreed rules the group could get out of hand. (Think of a sporting event with no rules: chaos!) All members should participate in establishing the rules at the first meeting, and a list of them should subsequently be displayed at meetings. New members should be given a copy of the rules on joining the group; they need either to agree with the rules or to propose amendments, which the group may accept or not.

Some examples of rules are:

- all members share the responsibility of group leader

- no members should be under the influence of alcohol or illicit drugs, or use them, during meetings
- confidentiality must be maintained about what is discussed: what is said in the group stays in the group
- all members should be on time for meetings
- members have the right to 'pass' (not to participate in a discussion)
- members will treat each other with respect

Agenda

Group members decide collectively on what topics should be discussed at meetings, and agree a format for them. Here is a sample agenda for a group meeting for two hours, between 10 a.m. and noon.

10.00 Welcome time, and to check with each member how they've been since the last meeting

10.20 Discuss the main topic of the meeting (allow members in rotation to present a topic for discussion, and then open it to all members to participate if they wish)

11.00 Break for 10 minutes for tea/coffee

11.10 Resume discussion, trying to ensure that all members get a turn to talk

11.50 Arrange next meeting: date, leader, topic

11.55 Close meeting, tidy up

If possible, allow time after the meeting for members to talk together informally for a while. There may be occasions when one member is in crisis, and the group needs to be flexible enough to give support even if it means changing the agenda. But there also need to be some boundaries: the group is not there to act as therapist for any individual member.

Different self-help groups evolve their own distinct character. What they all have in common is that they provide a safe environment for people to break their isolation and the pattern of feeling like a helpless victim: helping and being helped by people in the same situation as ourselves is very empowering. In the group it is possible to share experiences of the ways in which abuse has affected members' lives, and to offer mutual support during the healing journey.

APPENDIX 4

SELF-HELP RESOURCES

The following is a list of recommended books, audio tapes and videos.

General

The Courage to Heal, Ellen Bass and Laura Davis, HarperCollins, third edition, 1994

The classic, complete guide to healing for women survivors of child sexual abuse. This book is highly recommended by many survivors. The authors weave the personal experiences of survivors with professional knowledge and writing exercises in a compassionate and empowering book that offers invaluable support and guidance. The book maps out the healing journey and provides insights and strategies for partners of survivors, family members and counsellors. Bass and Davis obtained their information by interviewing many survivors who had been successful with their healing processes. The tone is calm, practical, hopeful and compassionate. This book is also available on audio tape.

The Courage to Heal Workbook, Laura Davis, HarperCollins, 1990

In this companion volume, Laura Davis provides checklists, open-ended questions, writing exercises, art projects and activities for men and women healing from the effects of child abuse. Ideal for use in self-help and group therapy.

Transforming Trauma: Treating Adult Survivors of Child Sexual Abuse, Anna Salter, USA, 1995

This book crosses the bridge between the experience of the victim and the psychology of the perpetrator. Salter answers the questions: What does the clinician who treats adult survivors need to know about sex offenders? And, how can trauma be not just endured, but transformed?

Breaking Free: Help for Survivors of Child Sexual Abuse, Carolyn Ainscough & Kay Toon, Sheldon Press, third impression, 1996

This book is primarily a self-help book compiled by two clinical psychologists. They draw on their experience and accounts of survivors to offer a book full of information and practical suggestions for overcoming the effects of abuse.

Emotional Abuse, Marti Tamm Loring, Lexington Books, 1994

This book provides a clear road map for therapists to guide them through the intricacies of treating emotionally abused victims. She describes both overt and covert emotional abuse and makes crucial linkages to other types of abuse as well.

The Drama of the Gifted Child, Alice Miller, HarperCollins, revised edition, 1994
Alice Miller is a psychotherapist who has written much about the negative after-effects of child abuse for both the individual and society as a whole. She pulls no punches and makes no excuses for perpetrators. In this revised version of her first book, she revises her theories in light of her own healing process and break with Freudian psychoanalysis. Be sure to get the revised 1994 edition of this book. Her other books include *Banished Knowledge: Facing Childhood Injuries, Breaking Down the Wall of Silence to Join the Waiting Child, The Drama of Being a Child, Thou Shalt Not be Aware: Society's Betrayal of the Child, For Your Own Good: The Roots of Violence in Child-Rearing*.

Making Sense of Suffering: The Healing Confrontation With Your Own Past, J Conrad Stettbacher, Penguin, 1991
In this popular book, psychotherapist Stettbacher provides the principles for his primal therapy as an effective way to resolve pain, and gives detailed information about his helpful 4-step process for working through memories of any kind of child abuse.

A Gift to Myself, Charles Whitfield, Health Communications, 1990
A gentle workbook on healing for adult children of dysfunctional families.

Memory and Abuse, Charles Whitfield, Health Communications, 1995
An excellent overview of the process of how childhood abuse affects the memory.

Healing Your Aloneness, Dr Erika Chopich & Dr Margaret Paul, HarperCollins, 1990
Offers some good advice about coping with the effects of child abuse.

Homecoming, John Bradshaw, Bantam, 1990
A classic guide to inner child work. Contains exercises and affirmations for every stage of development.

Toxic Psychiatry, Peter Breggin, St Martins Press, 1991
An important book about mis-diagnosis and mis-treatment in the mental health profession, especially how biological theories of mental illness are sometimes used to avoid dealing with social issues such as child abuse and domestic violence. Breggin makes some very important points about the dangers of biological psychiatry and abuses in the psychiatric profession.

Making Therapy Work, Fredda Bruckner Gordon et al, Harper & Row, 1988
An excellent guide to choosing a therapist and getting the most out of therapy.

A New Approach to Women and Therapy, Miriam Greenspan, McGraw-Hill, 1983
An important book on women's issues in therapy, which are sometimes overlooked or misunderstood.

My Precious Child, Mary Williams, Health Communications, 1991
A delightful book of inner child affirmations paired with beautiful photographs of children.

Once Upon a Time: Therapeutic Stories, Nancy Davis, Psychological Associates of Oxon Hill, 1990
A big book of warm, healing stories for both adult and child survivors of abuse. This book is not available in stores. To order it, write to: Nancy Davis, Psychological Associates of Oxon Hill, 6178 Oxon Hill Road, Suite 306, Oxon Hill, MD 20745, USA.

Putting the Pieces Together, Renee Fredrickson, Fredrickson & Associates, 1987
An excellent series of audio tapes on many different abuse recovery topics. Tapes can be ordered individually as well as in a complete set. For ordering information, write to: Fredrickson & Associates, 821 Raymond Ave, St Paul, MN 55114, USA.

Secret Survivors, E Sue Blume, John Wiley & Sons, 1990
A book on the adult after-effects of child sexual abuse. You're not crazy, you're a survivor! Highly recommended.

Shifting the Burden of Truth, Joseph & Kimberly Cornich, Recollex, 1992
An informative book on legal issues for adult survivors of childhood abuse.

When Ministers Sin: Sexual Abuse In the Churches, N & T Omerod, Millennium Books, 1995

Beyond Closed Doors: Growing Beyond An Abused Childhood, J Andrews, David Lovell Publishing, 1994

Recovery of Your Inner Child, Lucia Capacchione, Simon & Schuster, 1991
An excellent book of art therapy exercises for getting in touch with your inner child, including the left-hand/right-hand dialogue process many survivors have found helpful.

When Something Terrible Happens, Marge Heegaard, Woodland Press, 1991
This is a coloring book/activity book designed to help children work through trauma. The book is very helpful for little children.

Bessel A. van der Kolk: various excellent books, audio tapes and videos on coping with stress caused by abuse, for survivors and their families. Available from Guilford Publications, Inc, Dept. F, 72 Spring Street, New York, NY 10012, USA.

Repressed memories
Repressed Memories, Renee Fredrickson, Simon & Schuster, 1992
A validating, informative book on recovering and dealing with repressed memories. Highly recommended for any survivor who has recovered repressed memories.

Multiple personalities
Multiple Personality Disorder from the Inside Out, Barry Cohen et al, Sidran Press, 1991
An excellent collection of writings by multiples on various recovery issues. Highly recommended. Contains a chapter written by partners of multiples.

United We Stand, Eleana Gil, Launch Press, 1990
A simple, reassuring explanation of multiplicity. Good for people who have just been diagnosed, and for children.

The Family Inside—Working with the Multiple, Doris Bryant, Judy Kessler & Lynda Shirar, WW Norton & Company, New York, 1992
This book was written by two therapists and their client.

Ritual abuse
Safe Passage to Healing, Chrystine Oksana, HarperCollins, 1994
An inspiring, comprehensive guide for survivors of ritual abuse. Based on extensive research, in-depth interviews with survivors, and her own experiences as a survivor of ritual abuse. Oksana helps demystify ritual abuse cults and offers groundbreaking healing strategies.

Ritual Abuse—what is it, why it happens, how to help, Margaret Smith, HarperCollins, 1993
Smith examines the experiences of 52 adult survivors, cult abuse throughout history, the background of perpetrators, brainwashing and Multiple Personality Disorder. She gives compassionate guidance on the recovery and healing process.

Male survivors
Victims No Longer, Mike Lew, Cedar Publishing, 1988
A guide for men recovering from sexual child abuse. This book addresses male survivors with compassion and respect and helps them to identify and validate their childhood experiences, explore strategies of survival and healing, and work through issues such as trust, intimacy and sexuality. This is highly recommended as the best book for men by many ASCA members.

The Invisible Wound: A New approach to Healing Childhood Sexual Trauma, Wayne Kristberg, USA, 1993
Kristberg outlines a healing and recovery programme based on 'physical-energy blockages and body memories'. His Healing Journal includes more that a dozen techniques for self-exploration. The book also includes numerous personal stories of recovering survivors.

Abused Boys: The Neglected Victims of Sexual Abuse, M Hunter, Fewcett Colombine, 1990

Partners
Allies in Healing, Laura Davis, HarperCollins, 1991
When the person you love was sexually abused as a child. An excellent support book for partners and other significant loved ones, written in a question and answer format by one of the authors of *The Courage to Heal*.

Survivors tell their stories
Breaking Through, Cathy Ann Matthews, Albatross Books, 1990
Tells one victim's story and offers some practical steps to recovery. It was the subject of an award-winning film, shown on the ABC.

The Color Purple, Alice Walker, Pocket Books, 1992
A black woman documents her healing and growth process through her letter to God. A very realistic and inspiring novel.

Daddy, Please Say You're Sorry, Amber, CompCare, 1992
Amber hand lettered and illustrated her thoughts and feelings about her healing process in this delightful, powerful book.

Inside Scars, Sheila Sisk & Charlotte Hoffman, Pandora Press, 1987
A survivor and her therapist co-wrote this account of the survivor's healing journey. Contains actual therapy session transcripts.

The Obsidian Mirror, Louise Wisechild, Seal Press, 1988
Wisechild created an imaginary, symbolic world in which to play out her struggles to heal from incest. The book documents both her inner and outer journeys.

Scream Louder, Marsha Utain & Barbara Oliver, Health Communications, 1989
A survivor tells her story and her therapist highlights the issues being dealt with in this combination of self-help book/survivor's story. Lots of good information on dysfunctional families.

Step On a Crack, Pamella Camille, Freedom Lights Press, 1987
Vanessa, a funny, spunky survivor, tells her inspiring story.

Sex in The Sect, Vicky J, Essien, Melbourne
This book is a fascinating view into the mind of a multiple. To order the book, write to PO Box 2568, Bundaberg, Queensland 4670

TAKING LEGAL ACTION

'I have said ad nauseam on radio and television and in newspaper columns that the way our laws are structured in this country if you are a paedophile, the younger your victim the less chance of being caught, and if caught, the less chance of going to trial, and if charged the less chance of being convicted.

... It sounds brutal but what the courts are in fact saying to child molesters is: get them young and get them often. If caught, a molester's victim may not be allowed to testify against him. And if called, his (or her) evidence may be rejected on the grounds that they are too young or that their evidence is uncorroborated. And if you assault them often enough they won't be able to remember the exact date or times and their evidence will be discounted.'

Derryn Hinch, That's Life, *Penguin Books, 1992*

Making the decision
The decision to take legal action is a tough one in any situation. The legal process is not exactly renowned for its speed, clarity or ease for the average person. In the case of child abuse the decision can be much, much tougher.

An investigation into a crime requires details such as what clothes were worn by the parties involved, what time the crime allegedly occurred, where it occurred, and so forth. In the case of child abuse it often happened years ago, and on such a constant basis that it is difficult to pinpoint exact times, places and situations. The terror, shame and confusion a child feels at being hurt by someone they trust prevents the clear logical thinking that a legal case requires. Children often 'dissociate'—that is, they shut their mind off from what is happening—in order to cope with the immense distress they are enduring, so they may not even remember their abusive childhood until much later in life. This complicates matters further, as details such as what the perpetrator was wearing are of little or no significance to the victim. They remember the pain, horror, betrayal, shame, guilt, confusion, terror—an endless turmoil of emotions—but not the detailed facts necessary to bring a successful legal action.

The legal system as it currently exists relies on evidence to prove 'beyond reasonable doubt' that a crime occurred. The very nature of child abuse, however, is so covert, secret, concealed, that it is highly unlikely there will be any tangible evidence to show that the abuse has occurred. The perpetrator is most often someone known to the child—

either a member of the family or someone the child trusts—so he or she will try to keep the heinous, monstrous acts of abuse hidden for as long as possible (or, ideally for them, forever). Children do not have the resources to take themselves to the police, nor can they get away from the situation by getting a job and moving out. They are trapped in a horrible place. The perpetrator is usually either caring for them or is someone whom the carer trusts and/or loves. Perpetrators constantly tell their victims that no one will believe them, that it is their fault this is happening, and that they will destroy their family or be killed if they tell anyone. After this type of conditioning—which often goes on for years—it is unlikely that any evidence will be recorded by the child, and the abuser is certainly not going to help provide any evidence to prove his or her guilt.

This is not to suggest that anyone thinking of taking legal action should give up now. As you will have read in chapter 5, 'Breaking the Silence', survivors who have taken legal action have had both good and bad experiences with the legal system. Taking legal action can be enormously liberating for the abused person, because they finally and publicly take an 'official' stand against the terrible crimes committed against them, and they break the wall of silence that has kept them imprisoned for so long.

Examine your motives
What exactly is it that you want from a court hearing? Validation—that is, acknowledgment by society that you have been wronged? Punishment of the offender? Some compensation for what you have suffered? You need to be very clear about this.

If you desperately need the world to know that something awful really happened to you, the courts may be the last place to do this. Courts cannot decide what really happened. They have no way of doing this. They decide what has happened in law. Courts can provide some financial compensation (through the civil courts) and punish an offender (through the criminal courts) but you may not experience the process as validating. If what you need is to stand up and make yourself heard, the process, win or lose, may be enough. But if you need someone to acknowledge that your experience was real, maybe you should choose another way.

Going to court requires a lot of deep thought. But decide carefully what it is you want from it. We wouldn't complain if we couldn't buy apples in a hardware shop; we should be just enough not to demand that the courts give us what they do not have on offer or are not able to give.

Criminal and civil actions

The key to a successful court action is being as well prepared as you possibly can be. Some practical guidelines about the procedure follow.

Trials are either criminal or civil. The difference between them is not, as many think, a matter of greater or lesser degree of severity of the offence (rather like mortal and venial sins, for the Catholics among us), it is who brings the action. Criminal actions are brought by society (called the Crown) and civil proceedings are brought by private citizens. What you need to establish your case is also different. In criminal trials the offence must be proven 'beyond reasonable doubt', which is a very strict level of proof and means that there is no reasonable alternative explanation than the guilt of the accused. So if there is any such doubt, the case will not be made out. In civil matters it is 'on the balance of probabilities', which is an easier level of proof and merely means what it says: that on the balance of probabilities it is more likely than not the things complained of happened.

Much of the grief experienced by those who go to court is caused by a lack of understanding about what is involved. Legal practitioners are so used to their ideas, they lose track of what ordinary people do and do not know, and we, not knowing, don't know what to ask. Here are some of the differences between criminal and civil actions:

Criminal trial

Action brought by: the Crown (society).
Role of survivor: You will be a witness for the Crown, not a party, therefore you will not have your own barrister.
Level of proof required: Beyond reasonable doubt. This is a much tougher level of proof than is required in civil proceedings.
Possible outcome: Fines, jail terms, etc. That is, punishment of the convicted abuser, but not compensation for the survivor. It is society that is deemed to have been hurt, not the survivor.

Civil trial

Action brought by: the person harmed (an individual).
Role of survivor: You will be the plaintiff (the one bringing the complaint). You will have your own barrister.
Level of proof required: On the balance of probabilities, i.e. that it is more likely than not to have happened.
Possible outcome: Compensation is paid to the successful plaintiff, plus costs.

'Presumption of innocence'

It seems to us at ASCA that survivors face two sets of problems in going to court. One is that the legal system, which has been designed over a very long time to protect us in most legal situations, can seem like just more of the whole system of abuse when it comes to child abuse. It is designed on the principle that it is better for ten guilty men to go free than for one innocent one to be punished. So it does work to this end, and in most cases we would support that. It is just a different issue in the case of child abuse because in our experience the guilty always go free. We believe Australians need to think very carefully about what we value in the legal system, and what it is really telling us.

It is important for anyone contemplating legal action to realise that the 'presumption of innocence'—the supposition that the defendant is deemed to be innocent until proven guilty—is not a further abuse of you as someone who has already suffered, it is a vital part of our legal system, designed to ensure that the wrong people are not locked up. It can feel really bad, but it is part of what protects us in the normal course of events. Our courts try all offences, not just abuse cases. Think how you would feel if you had to prove that someone's accusations were false (that you'd stolen their video or damaged their car, for instance) instead of them having to prove them true.

What often also hurts is being 'just' a witness. People feel angry when they are told that they are not a party to the action. This does not mean that no one thinks they were not the primary person hurt, it just reflects that the case is being run by the Crown. So if the police charge someone, you will be a witness, not a party. In this case the offended party is 'society' and not you as an individual. This sounds as if it neglects the 'real' victim, but it is meant to signal that this is such an awful crime that it inflicts harm on the whole of our society and not just one person. It is, in fact, society standing up for us.

Taking action: what you will need

If you cannot date your allegation of sexual abuse to within six months of its occurrence, this will go against you in court. Being so certain of dates is often a very difficult task in cases of childhood sexual abuse because of the length of time that may have passed since the abuse occurred and the lack of surrounding landmark events that can help date the offences. The law also requires that the perpetrator be charged with specific offences rather than with ongoing behaviour. Thus the first step in deciding whether to take legal action or not should be to determine the accuracy with which events can be dated. It is not enough to say that the abuse happened when I was X years old at such and such an address. You will need to pin down the time of year and as much detail surrounding the assault as possible: what led up to it, what happened afterwards, etc.

You will need a degree of confidence and reasonable verbal skills. The court hearing is a battle of wits, and words are the weapons. Your words will be used against you in whatever fashion possible by the defence barrister during his cross-examination. The process of court action is very stressful and often frightening, and you will need a lot of support and practice in confronting the various issues. For this as well as for more general reasons, we at ASCA believe that it is advisable to be in regular therapy before, during and after the whole process.

It is vital that you come to your own decision about going to court. Therapists should not suggest this course of action to you, nor should they seek to dissuade you from it. You have to be clear about what happened and believe completely in your own memories and the meanings you attach to them, and not seek to have the court do this for you.

The first steps on the path to court
If you decide to proceed, the first step is to arrange for an interview with a detective from the Child Protection Unit of the Major Crime Squad. In some areas such units are not available, but you should make every effort to speak first to a detective experienced in these matters and skilled at relating respectfully to victims. Many people's experiences in these areas have been extremely positive, but there are also stories of people reporting sexual crimes to police and being blamed, disbelieved or treated unsympathetically.

The detective will want to take a statement from you and will want graphic detail, so you should be able to speak of these matters reasonably freely. Depending on the nature of the case, giving a detailed statement can take up to a full day. You can ask for as many breaks as you need, and it is quite acceptable to take someone along to support you.

The detective will type the statement and ask you to read and sign it. It is a good idea to take the statement away and read it later before you sign it, as however well prepared you are, you will still be in a state of some anxiety which may impair the thoroughness with which you read your statement.

The detective, in taking the statement, will have decided whether or not there is sufficient merit in your case to warrant an attempt at prosecution. If he or she has decided there is not sufficient merit, it is vital you realise that this means he has serious doubts the case would even get to court, let alone that the perpetrator would be found guilty. It does not mean he disbelieves your account of events. It is the detective's responsibility to ensure that only cases with some chance of being successfully prosecuted are processed further.

If he decides to proceed, he will forward your statement to the Director of Public Prosecutions, whose department acts as a second screen. There it will be reviewed, without you being present, by solicitors experienced in these matters. They will decide whether they believe that there is a reasonable chance of a successful prosecution. If they agree that the case is sound, the perpetrator will be arrested and charged with specific offences determined by the DPP. In most cases he or she will be bailed to appear in court at a date to be set for a committal hearing. It will commonly be some months between the DPP receiving your statement and this action being taken. The DPP proceeds with the majority of cases received, but once again, if they decline to proceed it means that they feel the case has little chance of success rather than that you are not telling the truth.

Committal hearings and arraignment hearings

A date for a committal hearing will be set, again generally many months after the perpetrator's arrest. This hearing is heard before a magistrate in a local court. You will not be required to be present unless you are called as a Crown witness. Your interests will be represented by the Crown prosecutor and a solicitor from the DPP, at no cost to you. Usually you will only meet these people a week or so before the trial. The perpetrator will be represented by his barrister at his expense, unless he is one of the few able to qualify for Legal Aid.

The committal hearing is to ensure that only those against whom a reasonably strong case can be made are put through a jury trial before a full court. For offences that occurred since about 1980, the perpetrator's barrister has been denied the right to cross-examine the victim. This change in proceedings was introduced so that such distressing evidence need be given only once. The perpetrator will generally be allowed out on bail, but will be required to be present at an arraignment hearing before a magistrate. This is the first opportunity the offender has to enter a plea of guilty or not guilty. There may then be a delay of anything up to 18 months before the case is heard in final detail.

At the trial there will be a jury unless the offender elects to have the case heard by a judge. Your interests will be represented by a barrister from the DPP, again at no cost to yourself. The perpetrator will be represented by his own barrister.

The process is undeniably stressful. If you feel up to it, taking legal action can be worthwhile. But, as with every aspect of recovery from abuse, it has to be your decision, your right, but in no way your obligation.

Some useful advice about going to court

From my own experience of taking my father to court I would like to make the following points:

- The decision to lay charges has to be the victim's. Once that decision is made, however, all further decisions about the conduct of the case are in other hands.
- Before making the decision whether or not to proceed, find out everything you can about the whole process: the taking of the statement by the police, the arrest procedure, bail conditions, the committal hearing, the trial, what support services are available.
- Ask any and as many questions as you like. It is about you.
- If you cannot work with the police officer/s assigned to your case, speak to the officer in charge and request a change.
- Request any available literature about the court process and read it through carefully.
- Make sure that you are informed of each stage in the process before it happens.
- If you feel the need for a screen to be placed in front of the perpetrator then demand it, and insist that every avenue is exhausted in trying to obtain it. It is your legal right to apply for it.
- If you want a support person with you during the whole process, that too is your right. Demand it. Rape/incest crisis workers are usually very good and very skilled at being support people.
- If you ever feel the need for protection from the accused, find out what can be done and demand it.
- Find out who in the prosecution's department is handling your case and contact them whenever you need to, recognising that there will be periods when they do not have additional information for you.
- If during the court hearings you feel like a break, ask for one. That too is your right.
- Keep a diary of everything that happens. Then you have a written account of what you have been told.
- Gather all the information you can regarding a criminal compensation claim.

Going to court is all about you, and you have the right to ask any questions, query anything, and demand whatever you are entitled to. Do not be swayed by someone saying you are not entitled to something. If you know for certain that you are, then insist.

My final piece of advice is to be prepared for the verdict to go either way. Be prepared, also, even with a guilty verdict, to be disappointed with the sentence imposed. I always concentrated on *why* I was doing it.

What I learnt from my court case

Since my court case ('the Bunbury case') in October 1994 I have learnt many things. I would like to share some of these with you. The following has been true for me:

- Depending on what is motivating you, the court process, though very painful, can be healing. It was for me.
- The court process is about the legal truth, not the whole truth.
- The media, in general, excel in getting the facts wrong! Journalists, with some honourable exceptions, seem more interested in a sensational story than in presenting the truth.
- What would seem to be a negative painful experience can in fact have positive aspects. There is always something we can learn and something we can grow from in all of life's happenings.
- It is better to feel the pain and let go of the grief, than to be bitter and harbour resentment.
- You cannot make another person listen. They will only hear you when they want to.
- The simple things in life are of the greatest value.
- I entered my healing process and the court case as a frightened little girl, and emerged as a woman.

Recent changes in the law

The laws surrounding the reporting of child abuse have changed in recent years. Here are two of the most relevant changes:

- Since 1986, it is no longer required under the law to have witnesses and/or other corroborating evidence in order to bring a charge of sexual abuse.
- Recovered memories: ASCA has been advised that, if a person's memories have not been recovered independently, then right from the outset that evidence will weaken the alleged victim's position in bringing about a charge of abuse. In the Director of Public Prosecution's view, independently recovered memories excludes the use of hypnosis, EMDR or any other 'overt' therapeutic intervention.

Getting help

If you do decide to take legal action, don't be embarrassed to ask for help. More than 1 in 5 people become a victim of crime or are indirectly affected by crime. Child abuse is one of the most horrendous crimes to endure, so support along the way is strongly advised. Ring your local Victims of Crime services (listed below), as they can provide:

- information about all services available
- supportive listening/counselling
- legal advice
- advice about support networks
- advice about court proceedings
- referral to grief and trauma counselling

New South Wales
VOCAL (Victims of Crime
   Assistance League)
02 9743 1636 (Sydney)
049 641 235 (Newcastle)

VOCS (Victims of Crime Service)
02 9217 1000
1800 819 816 (free call in NSW)
This is a 24-hour free counselling
   line

Police Customer Assistance
   Unit
1800 622 571 (free call)

Office of the Director of Public
   Prosecutions
02 9285 8949
1800 814 534 (free call)

   Compensation Court
02 9377 5444

Victims Compensation Tribunal
02 9375 6488

Witness Assistance Service
02 9285 8945

Salvation Army Counselling
   Service
047 311 554

Australian Capital Territory
VOCAL
06 295 9600

Victims of Crime Co-ordinator
   (Witness Assistance)
06 257 8452

Registrar of the Supreme Court
06 267 2707

Community Advocate
06 205 1075

Victoria
VOCAL
03 9655 5353

Crime Victim Services Geelong Inc.
052 253 100 or 041 110 1210

Crimes Compensation Tribunal
03 9628 7777 (Criminal Injuries)
03 9520 7511 (Magistrates Court)

Crime Victims Support
  Association
03 9761 0108

Witness Assistance Service
1800 641 927 (free call in Victoria)

DPP
03 9605 4333
1800 804 224 (free call in Victoria)

South Australia
Victim Support Service
08 8231 5626 or
  018 855 760

DPP
08 8238 2600
  (Commonwealth)
08 8207 1529 (SA)

Crimes Compensation Tribunal
1800 335 621 (free call in South
  Australia)

Injuries Compensation
08 8204 0287

Witness Assistance Officer
08 8207 5903

Queensland
There is no tribunal system in
  Queensland: the government
  grants ex gratia payments. These
  are usually handled by private
  solicitors or legal aid.

V.O.C.A. (Victims of Crime
  Association)
07 3221 7699

1800 640 840 (free call in
  Queensland)

Legal Aid Criminal Injuries
  Compensation Unit
07 3238 3462

Department of Attorney-General's
  Administration Law Division
07 3239 6975

DPP
07 3224 9444 (General)
07 3239 6840 (Victims of Crime
  Unit)
1800 673 428 (free call in
  Queensland)

Witness Information—Supreme and
  District Courts
07 3239 3331 (Brisbane)
07 3280 1716 (Ipswich)

Witness Information—Magistrates
  Courts
Enquiries to Queensland Police
  Service

Criminal Injury Compensation
07 3239 6546

Community Liaison Officer
  (Witness Assistance)
07 3239 6042

Western Australia
V.S.S. (Victim Support Service)
09 322 3711
1800 818 988
  (free call in WA)

The Assessor, Criminal Injuries
    Compensation
09 222 0210

Police Service
09 222 1111

DPP
09 264 1750

Child Victim Witness Service
    (Ministry of Justice)
09 425 2165

Tasmania
Attorney General's Department
03 6232 1700

DPP
03 6233 6649

Criminal Injuries Compensation
03 6233 3713

Victims of Crime Services
03 6228 7628 (Southern Tasmania)
03 6334 1665 (North Eastern
    Tasmania)
03 6431 9926 (North Western
    Tasmania)

Northern Territory
Attorney General's Department
08 8999 5511

DPP (including Victims Support
    Coordinator)
08 8999 7533

Aboriginal Legal Services
New South Wales
Aboriginal Women's Legal
    Service
02 9897 3168
Aboriginal Legal Service
02 9699 9277

ACT
06 257 6011

Victoria
03 9419 3888

South Australia
08 8211 8824

Queensland
07 3221 1448

Western Australia
09 265 6666

Tasmania
002 34 3955

Northern Territory
089 81 5266

Complaints to the Ombudsman

If for any reason you think you have been treated unfairly by a public authority or a public official (such as a member of the police force) you can complain to the Ombudsman for your state.

New South Wales
02 9286 1000
1800 451 524 (free call)

ACT
06 276 0111

Victoria
State: 03 9613 6222
Commonwealth: 03 9654 7355
1800 133 057 (free call)

South Australia
State: 08 226 8699
1800 182 150 (free call)
Commonwealth: 08 231 2861
1800 133 057 (free call)

Queensland
07 3229 5116

Western Australian
State: 09 220 7555 (general
  enquiries)
09 220 7568 (complaints against
  police)
1800 117 000 (free call)
Commonwealth: 09 220 7541
1800 117 000 (free call)

Tasmania
03 6234 9200

Northern Territory
Darwin: 089 81 8699
Alice Springs: 089 53 4933

APPENDIX 6

CANDIDA HUNT'S LETTER TO LIZ MULLINAR
This is the letter Candida wrote to Liz that supported Liz in her healing
and was the catalyst for the formation of ASCA.

Oxford, 20 September 1994

Dear Liz,

Lucy talked briefly about you to me today, and I can't ignore the urge
I feel to write to you. What follows is coming from my heart rather than
my head; if it evokes a response in yours, that will be fine, and if it
doesn't that will be fine too. I think it may.

The ideogram in Chinese for 'crisis' is composed of two symbols, that
representing 'danger' and that representing 'opportunity'. There is much
wisdom in this. It is so hard to welcome moments of crisis, when life
has always seemed a dangerous thing rather than an adventure. For you
and for me, danger has shadowed our lives. And we did not know; but
we knew.

A turning point for me was when I realised that I'd had a mistaken
view of myself in terms of courage. I had always felt ashamed and inadequate because fear held me back; then, when I found what I needed to
find—as you are doing—I discovered that so far from being feeble, my
survival and the ability to cope at all were demonstrations of great and
enduring courage. Honour the courage that has kept you going, and the
courage that has led you to find your truth.

There is a force for healing within us. We take it for granted when
we bruise our knees or cut a finger on a kitchen knife. But it is more
powerful and more profound than that. It has kept us going in ways we
have not been aware of and in spite of everything; it has led us to this
point, to the point where we are strong enough, mature enough, not to
be overwhelmed by the truth but finally to use this force knowingly, and
to release ourselves.

Do not be afraid. You will not be overwhelmed by what you find,
though as it comes closer this may seem to be likely. The healing force
that has protected you from the truth until you are ready to cope with
it will continue to protect you. You need do very little: allow it to
happen, provide time and space and safety for yourself, and when you
are ready, gradually let go … and it will come. It may be terrible; but
nothing you relive now will be as bad as the original experience, and
that you have survived. Admire the indomitable spirit of the child you

were, who survived, and has patiently waited all these years for a time when you are able to listen to her story, to comfort her, to accept everything she needs to tell you no matter how painful, how dreadful, how devastating . . . to release her at last from the secret she has carried. Only you can lift the burden from her, and when the time is right, you will.

Those of us who have had to spend our lives in hiding have experienced less love than we need. It seems to me that, for all the many shades of human emotion, really there are just two states: love and fear. They do not co-exist comfortably; the more of oneself that is burdened by fear, the less of oneself is available for love. I have found, as I release myself—and am released, for much of the healing takes place somehow on its own—from the fear that was once a way of life, that the capacity for loving (giving love and receiving it) grows. That is one of the lessons I have learned, and an important place to begin is with loving oneself.

Are you able to listen to yourself? I gave myself many a good talking to, listening was harder. Grown-ups tend to talk to (at) children rather than listening to what the children want to say, and trying to understand the reality in the child's perception. For me, another big shift came when I learned to shut up, and do no more than gather as much as I could of the quality of loving that I experience with my own children, and then try to bathe my child-self in the same love. It was difficult and awkward at first, but with perseverance I began to be able to trust myself more, and to listen more, and not to expect rational explanations (I am highly skilled at thinking away feeling when the feelings are painful and it's easier to rationalise them away than just to sit and feel them) or instant answers. I had to learn to take my time, to trust the wisdom that guides me towards healing. It's a lesson I have still not fully learned— old habits are hard to break.

Especially when the habits were once life-saving: like, never feel anger, because then I'd be in danger of remembering what I was really angry about, and that would have been perilous. But anger is the necessary power for self-protection, and without it you're a victim. Hard, too, to learn that being a victim is no longer inevitable. In the reclamation of onself that follows finding the truth, there are so many opportunities, so many discoveries to make—joy, spontaneity, a feeling of lightness that I think is 'not-fear' (and it wasn't, before, very easy to identify fear because there was never a state of not-fear, and we define things by the contrast their opposite provides), at times just a gladness.

The way of release from pain and fear is through the pain and the fear. It is the only way. Be patient, knowing that every little bit of pain you feel is another little bit released, another little bit you need never feel again. There are times to take the plunge; there are times to pause for rest and to gather strength. And all the time you will be leading yourself to the place where you need to be to tackle what you need to tackle, to find what you need to find. The loving innocence of the child you were before it happened, and the loving strength of the person you are now, together will embrace the hurt and frightened child who is waiting to be freed. There is joy as well as pain in the meeting, laughter as well as grief.

With all my heart I wish you well; the child I have rescued sends love, courage and faith to you and to yours.

In admiration,

Candida